Hospital Time

To Mary + Carol,
Love, Amy

HOS-
PITAL
TIME

AMY HOFFMAN

with a Foreword by Urvashi Vaid

Duke University Press   Durham & London   1997

© 1997 Amy Hoffman

Foreword © 1997 Urvashi Vaid

This edition © 1997 Duke University Press

All rights reserved

Printed in the United States of America on acid-free paper ∞

Designed by Deborah Wong

Typeset in Minion and Monotype Twentieth Century

by Tseng Information Systems, Inc.

Cover: Amy Hoffman, photo by Susan Fleischmann;

Michael Riegle, photo by Ellen Shub

Library of Congress Cataloging-in-Publication Data

appear on the last printed page of this book.

To Roberta, my heart

Contents

Foreword

Urvashi Vaid

Life with end-stage AIDS, like the struggle against any destructive illness, is not peaceful or pretty. Appropriately, neither is this unsettling memoir. In *Hospital Time,* Amy Hoffman details, without flinching, what it feels like to be responsible for a friend who is dying. From the middle of an experience most of us avoid at all costs and against a backdrop of far too many deaths, Hoffman constructs a sharp political memoir about the experience of lesbian and gay families in the time of AIDS. This insightful and disquieting book delivers a moving elegy on the quality of queer friendship, straight culture's abdication on AIDS, the meaning of mourning, and the possibility of redemption.

Mike Riegle was a friend of both Amy's and mine, so reading this book brought up many memories. Unlike Amy's "hospital time" with Mike, mine was limited by the convenient excuse of living in another city while his health declined. Unlike me, Amy and other friends mentioned in this book showed up every day to support Mike in his last two years of life. At the end of his life, no member of his family of origin came through for Mike. Mike had no lover, and even some of his best gay male friends stayed distant, pretending that he was as self-reliant as he had always been, acting as if AIDS changed nothing of his daily rituals and quality of life. Mike perpetuated that illusion—he was a stubborn, fiercely independent, proud man, who refused more than he accepted and eyed even friendly help with wariness and resentment.

The people who showed up for Mike were, like Amy, members of his lesbian and gay family. In describing this truth directly, without didacticism, this book points out the tremendous expansion of the idea of traditional family that lesbian and gay people have effected, an expansion that AIDS further cemented. And Hoffman's book suggests questions that gay and straight people have yet to answer. How did a people so ostracized by an institution end up reinventing it? What does the concept of family mean to a people so starkly abandoned by our traditional families of origin? Given the complete rejection by so many parents of gay people, siblings, aunts, uncles, cousins, and others who by tradition and obligation are "supposed" to be there for us, why do we continue to give places of honor to nuclear family members who never came to visit our friends during the many long, harsh months and years of their decline? Why do we keep on loving and forgiving these families when they hurt us so badly?

Family is an overused and politicized term in American life today and has been especially since the late 1970s when the Right discovered that calling someone anti-family was as potent as calling him or her a communist. As Gore Vidal writes, "Since hardly anyone ever openly questions the value of the family in human affairs, any group that wants to save this allegedly endangered institution is warmly supported."[1] Sometimes the notion of family values is proposed nostalgically, to hide the postindustrial deterioration of family ties and commitment. At other times, the concept serves to divide and conquer, demarcating the line between "real" (read nuclear) families and "fake" ones (gay, feminist, unmarried, single-parent). Most often, the idea of family is presented as static and absolute, as if the institution remains unchanged by the economic, cultural, gender, legal, and political revolutions of the past century. The truth differs from this myth. The nature, power, and roles of families change dramatically as the economic forces that govern our lives change. And, in fact, the force most responsible for transforming today's "traditional" families is not feminism nor gay and lesbian liberation, but capitalism. For example, it was the mobility brought on by industrialization and wage labor that allowed people to move to cities or move for jobs far away from the farms or communities in which they had extensive family ties — thus weakening the traditional bonds of family and geography.

Throughout the short history of modern gay and lesbian community, anti-gay prejudice and cultural ostracism have been the constants. These pressures placed on gay friendships and gay institutions roles and duties that for most heterosexuals are fulfilled by their traditional families. For gay people, our friends form our nuclear families, while our communities take on the role of an extended family system. And during the traumatic times of caring for each other during the multiple epidemics of AIDS, cancer, violence, youth suicide, and homophobia that we face, our alternative family structures proved themselves to be as solid and formidable as traditional families are for heterosexual people.

There are undeniably thousands of parents and siblings who have cared for their gay loved ones living with AIDS and HIV. Strong leadership has been shown by Mothers Against AIDS, Parents and Friends of Lesbians and Gays, and similar organizations. But it is also true that in the lives of most gay and bisexual men, this family never shows up. Their fear of AIDS expresses itself as too little, too late—like the brother who arrives at Mike's memorial service after the gay family has taken care of all the messy details. As Hoffman writes, "The healthy brother, he turns up with his man-of-the-family authority draped about him like a red scarf, and we kowtow to him like deformed trolls living under a bridge to one who walks in the light. The real family doesn't have to do anything. . . . With AIDS, nine times out of ten, it's the fake family who cleans up the shit."

Reading these sentences brought back the memorial services I have attended where AIDS is never mentioned and the twin services, one for the gay family and the other for the straight. Who among us has not sat through the memorial service in which the traditional family arrives—tearful, entitled, sometimes penitent—to claim a place at the end of a life which they earlier abdicated? Hoffman's memoir evoked for me the scores of instances I know in which mention of the surviving lover was erased in the tradition-ridden rituals of mourning, which still make no place for gay people. It reminded me of my disorientation at hearing a friend's wrenching struggle to maintain a decent quality of life—in the midst of medical uncertainty, physical pain, dementia, and hideous psychic torment—recast after his death as a noble or spiritual battle, rather than as the debasing, desperate, horrible clutching for life-at-any-cost it was.

Hoffman's book bears quiet witness to the emergence of gay and lesbian families during this time of AIDS. In fact, gay men and lesbians are in the middle of a creative revolution in family-creation, marked by the commitment we have shown in caring for each other, the expansion of child-bearing, and the centrality to us of our relationships and friendships. Without sermons or government orders enforcing our duty to care for each other, gay and lesbian people have invented a network of organizations and institutions to care for each other; we have built community centers, health organizations, service organizations, support groups, and political organizations, all with a minimum of public funds and in the face of great cultural hostility. More of us are becoming parents, choosing children through adoption, foster care, alternative insemination. Relationships—of the committed as well as the purely sexual kind—have a priority in gay life that puzzles heterosexual people. Our family commitment to each other is not forced, but desired; our marriages are not arranged for economic benefit or social duty; our children are chosen and beloved, not incidental and taken for granted.

What surprises me in our political movement is that we fail to see that embracing the idea of family does not mean we are reproducing it in gay drag: we are not reproducing family in just the same way that our parents did. In failing to talk about the ways we have broadened the meaning of family beyond the dyad of mom and dad into friendship, we gloss over some of the wonderful and unique differences we have—which make our relationships more equal than our parents' relationships ever were, which make our children more tolerant and healthy and aware than we ever were, which make our community's response in the AIDS epidemic so extraordinary. In fact, gay families and gay relationships are wonderfully and refreshingly different from straight families. For example, gay parents involve their friends and community in the process of coparenting and raising our children far more than many heterosexual parents. Amy goes every Wednesday to spend time with her best friend Betsy's daughters. Two other lesbians are planning to have a child with a close gay male friend, and all three will raise the baby. Another lesbian friend who is single shares custody with the child's gay father, who lives in an apartment above hers. These conscious, chosen arrangements have few corollaries in the traditions of the middle-class nuclear family. In many ways, our queer families bear a closer resemblance to the traditional extended families of many ethnic groups and are similar to the shared parenting relationships necessary for survival in working-class and poor families, where economic realities necessitate a community of support and interdependence. By expanding the role of friendship into family, gay and lesbian people offer the static and decaying heterosexual families of our time the possibility of saving the love—the soul—that underlies the obligation.

My queer family is vastly bigger and broader than my biological family. It includes friends in different cities, like Amy and Mike—a network of men and women, gay and straight, who take care of me, shelter and assist me in every way, and would give all they had to help me, if I needed. It is this queer family to whom I turn—on a daily basis—for comfort, advice, and support. This family of queer friends is the one with whom I share my daily joys and trials. We commiserate or brood about the struggle for economic survival. We loan each other money and talk about how we want to save for things in the future. We work together in the movement. We cook each other dinner, make sure we have soup when we have the flu, walk each other home late at night, call up and make sure we are okay, mourn our friends and the passing of relationships. My queer family loves me and knows me in a way that my heterosexual family, as close as it is to me, with its formal forays into my life on the ritualized occasions of holidays, ceremonies, and family gatherings, never will. It is this queer family that *Hospital Time* makes visible.

To read this book is emotional because Amy Hoffman is such a clear and honest writer. We witness scenes that propriety and tradition deem open only to certain kinds of people—spouses, lovers, mothers, and other family members. We feel Hoffman's anger at her helplessness as she watches parts of her history, her own life, die with the bodies of her gay male friends. We share Hoffman's fury at Mike's obstinacy, we listen to her self-doubt, we squirm at the honest, unanswerable questions of whether she is doing the right thing in deciding—as Mike asked her to do—whether doctors should use extraordinary measures to save his life or let his body's weakness take its course.

Hoffman writes of the details of end-stage AIDS—layering the experience of decline in the frustrating, haphazard way it happens, rather than glossing it over with abstract digressions on the metaphysics of dying. She vividly shatters the helpful but inaccurate political euphemism we have created to comfort us—that of people "living with AIDS"—to expose the shit-stained truth of wasting bodies, open sores, pain, shame, homophobia, and the maddening passage, minute by minute, of hospital time.

In the end, this book's impact comes as much from the political context of AIDS as from its powerful language. Fifteen years into an epidemic that has claimed more than 400,000 American lives, people in the communities most affected struggle to prevent new infections without government support.[2] Despite the fact that hundreds of thousands of people live with AIDS and HIV infection today (estimates hover at one million), mainstream culture in 1996 continues a pattern of denial and personal rejection toward people with AIDS. Our culture's denial of AIDS expresses itself in overwhelming political silence and personal absence on the part of our families of origin, a silence that is mirrored by mainstream politicians, hypocritical organized religion, and fickle media attention. That this epidemic continues to be so pervasive and so denied, so painfully immediate to literally millions of Americans and so fastidiously unaddressed in "polite" mainstream conversation is the ongoing tragedy that frames *Hospital Time.*

More than two-thirds of all people who have died of HIV and AIDS in the United States so far were gay or bisexual men. Two-thirds of 400,000 is 266,000. This is more than the number of Americans killed in any modern U.S. war. More than the number of American soldiers remembered in all the U.S. war memorials except those from the Civil War. Line up the bodies in graves, and you would nearly fill Arlington National Cemetery. Mike Riegle would have hated any comparison between AIDS and war. I can hear him chastising me, "Really, you could be less trite. That war metaphor is such a cheap way to sanctify gay worth. Like we need to justify ourselves to them."

Mike hated to be compared to any aspect of a dominant culture he considered bankrupt. Yet how are we to make visible these massive deaths, huge losses of cherished friends, picked off one by one?

The gay community has developed rituals, codes, structures, and institutions that strangely normalize the horror of life with this epidemic. These community responses combine a form of self-protective denial (acting as if we have the fire under control) and self-loathing acceptance of this epidemic as inevitable (a response disclosed recently by activists studying attitudes toward AIDS among young gay men).[3] Courageously, Hoffman rejects both the gay denial and gay acceptance of the inevitability of AIDS. Her hatred of AIDS is the anger of a veteran present at too many body counts. Her response — to show up, shoulder her responsibility as a friend, stay courageous and willing to love — describes the heroism of ordinary lesbians and gay men who move ahead with life from the center of so much death.

Notes

1 Gore Vidal, "Sex Is Politics," reprinted in *United States: Essays 1952–1992* (New York: Random House, 1993), p. 543.

2 Amanda Bennett and Anita Sharpe, "AIDS Fight Is Skewed by Federal Campaign Exaggerating Risks," *Wall Street Journal,* 1 May 1996, p. A1.

3 See Walt Odets, *In the Shadow of the Epidemic* (Durham: Duke University Press, 1995); Eric Rofes, *Reviving the Tribe: Regenerating Gay Men's Lives in an Ongoing Epidemic* (Haworth Press, 1995).

Introduction

Hospital Time

In Intensive Care a clock hangs on the wall opposite the bed. Big black numerals. One hand that moves in sudden ticks, minute by fucking minute.

The better places put up a calendar as well, although its usefulness is debatable when you think about it, since intensive care patients aren't exactly able to wander over and cross off each day at bedtime, before toothbrushing. They're sleeping and waking at random, and the primal distinctions—"And it was day and it was night and God saw it was good"—all that's long gone. So how are they supposed to orient themselves in relation to a calendar illustrated with a photograph of the snowcapped Alps? The nurses could cross off the days for the patients, but they don't; perhaps they think it would be tactless, too emphatic of the constant slippage of the present into the swamp of the past until that red-letter day when it's sucked down into it forever by you-know-what. And we visitors are intimidated by all of the tubes and wires and monitors that hook up to machines that are hissing, sucking, clicking, chattering, and we're afraid to deface hospital property. What would the date mean, anyway, in that place?

The hour is another story: there are dosages of painkillers to wait for. There are also tortures—whoops!—treatments to endure: the tube down the throat or up the nose, the needle in the neck or the spine, the catheter, those are treatments, and a clock doesn't help with those. There's no end in sight to treatment, or at least you hope not, so you don't want to know the time. Five minutes gone; if you're lucky, or if you're not, five zillion to go.

Time ticks by differently next to the sickbed. Nothing's happening—or maybe it's everything that's happening, or is about to. And there's no comfortable place to sit. The bed is narrow, the patient

3

bristling with needles, electrodes, and other ICU accoutrements that must not be displaced. I've been reading up on accounts of terminal illness; often visitors resort to massaging the feet, the only place on the body where contact is unimpeded.

I sat on the edge of Mike's bed or on a stool or chair next to it and cupped my palm around his shoulder. Sometimes I held his hand, but often it was swollen from the IV taped into the back of it, and a blood oxygen monitor was clamped to one finger. We would speak, when he was able. He would ask for things, and I would get them. Or we would sit in silence, and I'd wonder if I should say something. Something profound, something appropriate to this most profound of situations.

"How are you doing?"

No answer.

My neck would begin to ache, then my buttocks. My arm would fall asleep. I'd think of obligations elsewhere. I'd get bored. I'd wish I'd brought a magazine to look at. A magazine! Mike was struggling, he was dying, and he needed my total attention. My total palm on his shoulder.

Some people believe in the laying on of hands, and they're not all religious fanatics either. Look at Mike's friends. Look at Loie, coming to visit Mike in the ICU at Beth Israel. She took his hand, and then she demonstrated t'ai chi for him—no sitting around on the bed for her. She stepped back into the room away from the monitors and began to move slowly over the linoleum. "The monkey . . . the swan . . . pushing back the clouds," she explained, eyes closed. Her hands traced patterns in the air. Mike's eyes were closed too. He lay on his back facing the ceiling, his bony nose jutting like a monument out of his emaciated face. Air rushed and gurgled through his oxygen mask. In the hallway, the nurses ignored us, but the doors to rooms in the ICU are never shut, the curtains never entirely closed. I was aware that we might look ridiculous.

I would shift my position slightly, and Michael would say, or not say, but I knew he was thinking, "Leave, if you want."

"No," I'd say. "I'm fine."

I'd set goals: to stay until I'd helped Mike eat his lunch, until the nurse came to change the bed, until the doctor and his entourage kicked me out. Nothing happening. Everything happening. The minutes would tick by, stretch by, leap by, poke by, and I'd fluff up the pillows, demand another blanket to tuck around Mike's feet—he hated for anyone to see his feet, thought they were terribly ugly—fetch the bedpan or a cup of juice and a straw.

The patient lies in the ICU, and you charge in gabbing about the weather, which you have brought into the room: you shake the rain from your hair, or the cold air reddens your cheeks and clings to your coat, or sweat beads on your upper lip and dampens the hair on your temples. You draw the patient's attention to the view from the window, the time of day: the sun, the moon, the clouds. Your vigor, your life outside, is an affront. It's utterly frivolous, the world and its stupid times. Here in the hospital is the real thing. Eternity.

Living with AIDS

Distractions

I hated myself during the era of Michael's sickness. I pushed myself into the middle of it, and then I not only resented him and his needs and his crazy demands, but I also became jealous of anyone else who took care of him, who stopped in for a visit even. I wanted to be better than all of them.

And I was worse. People would say, "You're wonderful to do so much for him," and I'd feel they'd exposed my hypocrisy. For example, Fran called me last night. She and Stephanie miss Michael and often talk about him.

I don't. And I don't miss him.

They want to get together with me so we can all talk about him. Fran said she drives by his building and looks up at his window. The lights are on; there's a new tenant. Actually, I knew that. I've driven by his building and seen those lights, too. My theory is that it's the guy who lived in the tiny studio next door, Frank or something. Mike had a one-bedroom. It's okay, Frank deserves to move up in the world, a sweet, bubbleheaded young thing who worked out a lot at the gym so that when we were clearing all the junk out of Mike's apartment he was able to be very helpful lugging boxes of papers and bags of trash down the stairs.

Frank wanted to help me carry the air conditioner, which I had forced Michael to buy during the summer's heat wave—I took him shopping at Lechmere for it. Imagine that—Michael in the appliance department, walking slowly down the aisles as though every step pained him, and of course it did, his neuropathy, but also he ached with disapproval of all that *stuff*. It worked out, we bought the thing, but only because the salesman was Italian. At one time Mike had lived in Italy; he spent his years there adoring the Italians—their

9

dark sexiness, their emotionalism, their anarchist politics. The salesman was a middle-aged Sicilian who unbuttoned his shirt to show us the scar from his heart surgery. He couldn't take the heat either.

I didn't want help from Frank or anyone else. I wanted to carry the air conditioner down the stairs with superhuman strength. By the time I got it out to the car I was faint, and I had to rest for a moment on the front stoop of the building, head between my knees, as Mike himself must often have done. I haven't unloaded it yet either. It's in the back seat, but I'm not worried; it's too fucking big to steal, and it's only April. The heat's still on.

Frank even let us into his place to use the phone. For all I know, he isn't bubbleheaded at all. I think I heard something about medical school. Maybe he thought that if he was nice to us he'd have a better shot at Mike's one-bedroom apartment, not that we had any particular clout with the landlady. I'm sure Mike refused to have anything to do with Frank the whole time they were neighbors, as nice as Frank was, sticking his head out the door all the time and offering help, and Mike would have gotten all pissy about our inviting him in and allowing him to get involved with Mike's personal boxes. He would have sulked in the corner like a ghost, refusing even to say hello, and I would have had to chatter away to Frank so he wouldn't feel completely unwelcome. Mike would have disapproved righteously of Frank, and after Frank left he would have abused him for spending his time on something as trendy, vain, and politically irrelevant as working out at the gym, not to mention going to medical school. When the reality under all Mike's sulking would have been that it was he, not I, who wanted him there.

Frank was too cute. He was a distraction.

I knew Michael the same way I know just about everyone I'm close to in my life: he and I worked together at *Gay Community News* years ago. It was quite a time—the late seventies, no AIDS. None. I was the managing editor and Mike was the office manager, and here's a story: once we got a student intern from the University of California. Scott—I still see his byline in the gay press from time to time. He wrote us a card, and then one day he showed up in the office.

Shoulder-length blond hair, bright blue eyes, muscles, a tan. A real California surfer. I'd learned enough about gay men by then to think immediately when he walked in: "This is trouble." The office would be buzzing for weeks with all kinds of intrigue, rivalry, drama, no one getting any work done—when they were supposed to be training the kid, not seducing him. Sure enough, soon there was Scott, sitting on Mike's lap. But later, Mike told me angrily to keep Scott away from him, away from his desk, away from his whole side of the office. He didn't want to know he was around. He demanded I send him back to California. Like it wasn't a free country, and Scott couldn't be an intern and a flirt if that was what he wanted. Mike denounced him: he was a *distraction*. So, it wasn't only the HIV that brought out that desire and fury in him.

Distraction.

I can hear Michael say it, in that deep voice of his, which people always, *always* asked about if he called me at work, even straight men. I could've put money on it: "Who is that guy with the sexy voice?" It was remarkable. If they only knew. Michael, in his rags. He patched his clothes himself, but not neatly, since he didn't believe in that. On his favorite shirts the thread was stronger than the fabric, so it frayed rather than mended them, and the colors never matched. A seamstress he wasn't, but he was terrifically proud of his lousy work. Often he didn't bathe, and he didn't do much laundry, either. This was before he got sick. It had nothing to do with weakness or fatigue. Cleanliness, sanitation—he believed these were bourgeois affectations. It was a political position. The native Americans, I used to want to point out to him, were bathing daily when the Europeans thought immersion would kill you. He was interested in anthropology and of course in deferring to the leadership of indigenous peoples. But I didn't want to be rude, and I could think of no way of acknowledging his body odor with humor or tact; *rude* was a word of his, he used it a lot.

Michael often smelled, and I, bourgeois that I am, never liked to touch him. He wasn't a touchy person—I'm not either—so maybe he didn't notice. Occasionally, when we were leaving each other, we'd stand side-by-side, and he'd give me an awkward squeeze around the shoulders, but usually I just waved foolishly at him, fluttering my fingers. His answering wave was dignified—a quick jerk of his open hand to the side. "*See ya.*" In that voice.

One evening, when he was on the respirator, he made me lie down in bed with him. I didn't understand what he wanted at first. And of course he couldn't talk. He had to write everything on a yellow pad on a clipboard that was labeled "Respiratory Crisis Communication Aid Device" or something insane like that, although it was nothing but the most ordinary of clipboards, worn away and cracked along the bottom. By the end of the day it had become such a strain that his penmanship was all shaky, and he was writing one line on top of another. He couldn't see straight. I was proposing all sorts of things—"Do you want some water? A painkiller? Should I get the nurse?"—and finally he grappled my head down to his chest, and I lay there stiffly, the intensive care nurses peering at us through the door, until his arms around me relaxed in sleep. They all thought I was his wife anyway. It happened one other time after that, the night I stayed over at his house, but he didn't have to force me then. He wanted comfort, as anyone would, and I thought, "I had set my limit at this, but we're way past the world of reasonable limits now," so I tried my best to lie beside him calmly and generously.

Frank. Michael resented encountering healthy, vigorous, sexy men. They aroused him, yet toward the end, the last six months or so, even before that, he had lost the emotional and physical strength for arousal. It would make him furious: he never lost the energy for that. He felt they were rude, parading around in front of him. The beach in Provincetown made him literally sick. He shouldn't have been out there in the hot sun, but he insisted, when anyone would have known what it would be like. There are places back in the dunes, when the tide comes up, where I've happened upon flocks of men floating naked on inflatable toys in the warm tidepools. It's like a porno movie, only not grainy or sordid, but sunwashed and kind of sweet. Mike had some fantasy of what would happen to him back there, and it overrode what little good sense he had.

Here's another fantasy of Mike's: Pointing out a guy rolling down the street, he told me he wanted to find a boyfriend in a wheelchair.

With such a person he wouldn't have had to feel ugly or emaciated. He would take care of him.

Michael was brilliant, no question, spoke three or four languages, played the piano by ear, but what an idiot he was. He thought he was taking care of himself so well he was ready to move on to others. He never shook that fetish for the paternal role. Finding a young man on the street and reforming him. Advising, providing, fucking him up the ass until the boy spoiled it all by ripping him off or getting drunk and hitting him over the head. Michael never figured out what all of us who appeared around him were doing there. Why he needed us. At least, he never acknowledged it, never thanked anyone. Quite the opposite.

I tried to think daily about Maimonedes. In Hebrew school we wrote in blue notebooks with a picture of him in his turban on the cover. Hundreds of years ago he was a doctor in Spain, and the Jews are still proud of him. He wrote that there was a ladder of charity with eight rungs. At the bottom rung, you ask me for something; I give it to you. Nu? It's good enough for most people, but the righteous work their way up to the higher rungs, where the interactions are unsolicited and anonymous. At the top, giver and receiver have no knowledge of one another. The ego of the giver, her desire for the indebtedness, the enthrallment, of the receiver, never enters in. I agree with Maimonedes about this; he knew that gratefulness would not keep us taking care of one another. The recipient of your gift doesn't want what you've given, or wants more, or doesn't recognize that you've given anything at all.

Michael didn't thank me, or anyone. He might talk enthusiastically about one friend to another, but never directly to that person. Like the time he refused to speak to Jenifer in the car on the way home from their weekend in the country. She took him to visit a lesbian writer well-known in certain radical circles with whom Jenifer, notoriously nonmonogamous, was having an affair. The affair included the writer's lover, also. To everyone else Mike raved about this visit, speaking in an especially sycophantic way about the writer's home and her attentions to him, so that anyone hearing him felt she couldn't possibly give him anything nearly as precious as what

Jenifer had given. And Jenifer had genuinely wanted him there. She invited him without second thoughts, without regrets, at least until he turned on her. So it's true that I, at least, could never have given him anything like that. If I were Jenifer, I would've resented his presence, the demands on my attention taking me away from my exciting new lovers. Jenifer herself heard none of Mike's ravings about their trip. She thought he was angry at her, and she was hurt. She could think of no reason for it. And maybe he was.

He did say one thing to me the night I stayed at his apartment. It was his last night at home before the final time he went into the hospital. I didn't want to stay over, but I had to. Others had already taken their turns cheerfully. I didn't want to sleep at his place. I didn't want to cover myself with his scratchy pilled blankets and clammy sheets. I didn't want to use his filthy bathroom in the morning, or his coffee cups. But he couldn't stay in his apartment alone — we had all agreed about that — and there was no place else for him to go. Not that he wanted to leave. Didn't see the need. The view from his bedroom window of sky and the trees of the Fenway was one of his final pleasures.

Diarrhea kept him up all night. He wouldn't call for help, but I would wake when I heard him crashing around. His body wasn't telling him anything anymore, and when he would finally realize what was happening, he wasn't strong or quick enough to get himself across the narrow hall to the toilet. He refused to use the adult diapers we had bought or the bedside commode we had ordered. Maybe he associated the commode with intensive care. Although there, he'd insisted on the commode; the nurses wanted him to stay in bed and use a bedpan, but they didn't always come when he called. So he'd struggle up to find the toilet, and when they finally arrived they'd find him collapsed on the floor. Eventually they tied him to the bed, and I had to get the chaplain to intercede. Mike promised to behave after that, and they brought in the commode as a reward. I spent the night I stayed at his apartment cleaning off his bum when he didn't make it, mopping shit off the floor, and helping him in and out of the bathtub. After each episode, he'd doze off briefly, then it would start all over: I'd hear something, Michael standing in the bedroom doorway, moaning, shit spewing from his behind as from a monster in a Boschian Hell. The mop, the bath. Toward morning, he told me it was the best night he'd had in months. "This is how I live," he said. "No one knows what I go through. The others didn't help me clean. They didn't wake up." He asked me to lie down beside him until he fell asleep. "Your presence is a comfort," he said. "I'd say it was your aura, if I believed in things like that." He laughed his low laugh.

"Thanks," I said. It was the only time I felt that I was doing right after all—after all my doubts, all his complaints. I cherish it, although it's not pure. I know the others helped, and without my petty discomforts and resentments. He didn't have to deny them.

A million times I tried to analyze my jealousy. I had vowed to take care of him, and I fulfilled that vow. With the virus, you make a choice. When someone gets sick, you're either in or out. That's it. No middle ground. I visited Mike at *Gay Community News* when he first started getting the fevers—he was still working there after twelve years, unlike me, he never quit—and I took his hand and told him he could call on me any time. It was an impulse, sitting together in this dark little cave of an office he'd constructed for himself at the back of the building, but I was serious, although he didn't take me seriously at the time. He wasn't really paying attention—his fever was going up. I once heard a show on National Public Radio about kidney donors. When the doctors called the potential donors, they responded instantly: "Okay. Sure." Or else: "Nope." Astounded, the doctors asked them didn't they want to think it over? They said "What for?" That's exactly how it happened to me. There's nothing to think over when you're confronted with a decision like that: yes, you do it; no, you don't.

Later, Mike asked me to be his healthcare proxy, to make decisions in case he couldn't, and we went to his doctor to discuss it. I showed the doctor a chart that I'd sent away for from the American Medical Association that listed catastrophes across the top—"in a persistent vegetative state," "brain damage and terminal illness," "brain damage and no terminal illness," etc.—and treatments down the side— "cardiopulmonary resuscitation," "mechanical breathing," "chemotherapy," etc. I thought the doctor would find me an exceptionally well-prepared and thoughtful proxy, but he looked at the chart impatiently. "You can't possibly anticipate every eventuality. It's more important to talk about this together, so you understand how Mike thinks."

That'll be the day.

Obediently, I tried bringing it up a few times, but Mike wouldn't let me steer our conversations in that direction. We often talked long and deeply, but about topics that Michael introduced. These were wide-ranging, but dying wasn't among them. Age, yes. Loss of youth and beauty, yes. Infirmity, yes. But not the persistent vegetative state. In the end, Mike left me twisting in the wind.

Because he didn't want to bother anyone. *That* was how he thought. I would check on him each day or two, but rarely did he call me without any prompting, unless something had set him off and made him feel exceptionally lonely. He'd tell me he longed for a lover. He'd sigh and flutter his hand over his chest, although of course he pushed away any potential lovers. And they did appear, until nearly the end. Peter was one. Mike banished him from his life, keeping only a huge blob of a cactus plant, spiny and hideous, that Peter had given him. There was also the New Yorker who wanted to take him on romantic weekends to the Cape. Maybe they were too old for him, too close to his own terrible age, which was old enough, yet also so young and unfair. But he also spurned a boy who latched onto him at the newspaper. The boy gave him a blowjob, and then, seeing the stars in the boy's eyes, Mike said he'd only been interested in the sex. He surrounded himself with women like me and a few mumbling men with untended beards. They were gay, but they lacked that gay grace, instead *shlepping* their bodies around like they were taking out the garbage.

Then came Timo — a straight boy with long hair and an Asian girlfriend — Michael's last, his greatest distraction.

The two were new members of a group Mike had belonged to for years that gathered each week in the basement of a socialist bookstore to mail books and other information to prisoners. Coyly, Mike would pat Timo when Timo walked by him with a stack of prisoners' letters. He would bump against him on their way out the door. Surely Timo had caught on. The question was whether he felt even a faint glimmer of interest. The whole thing repulsed me, Mike's sleazy advances to young men. His dignity abandoned, his powerful desires broken into meek, greasy half-gestures. Mike felt guilty about the Asian girlfriend, not liking to interfere with the relationships of a woman of color deserving of his respect.

It was one of Mike's better days, and we were taking a walk around the pond near my house. People bursting with health passed us carrying fishing rods, jogging, rollerskating, biking. Park police trotted by on horses. We shambled along for a few hundred yards and then sat down on the bank to rest, and Michael told me of his longing. He was tremendously agitated about a dream he'd had in which Timo requited his love. So did the Asian girlfriend; it seemed only polite to let her into it, too. The dream left him feeling greatly hopeful; it was a portent. He wondered what I thought: should he say anything? After all, there was the girlfriend, and Timo's clear sexual preference. But how clear was clear? Mike had had plenty of straight trade in his life, in the bushes, in the tearooms, in the baths. He'd been one of them himself for a time — although not a time that he talked about. Was that the message of his dream — that nothing was clear, all was layered and murky? When I was in elementary school the science teacher had brought in a mica rock that peeled apart in layers that you could see through. But you could not see through the rock.

Mike told me his plan: He would pull Timo aside at the organization's next potluck. It was the coming weekend. He would ask Timo to chastely lie with him. He would ask only for comfort. He would humble himself and abjectly beg for comfort. He would cite his age, his ugliness, his pitiful illness, and Timo, if he had a heart, would not turn him away.

But does a straight boy have a heart? Timo rebuffed him and after that skirted him widely in the bookstore basement, keeping far from Michael's sneaking hands. What must he have thought? To have been groped by those plague-stricken hands, the emaciated arms of death stretching toward him from the boiling Pit, stretching toward comfort, toward love. Terrified Timo flees. He avoids his girlfriend's welcoming kiss, runs to the shower where his tears mingle with the scalding drops of water. He can't make love to her for a few days, but then in a rush of pain he wants it again. Their healthy orgasms are sweet, so sweet.

Timo and his girlfriend joined the parade of people in and out of Mike's hospital room. They made a crayoned sign on a big piece of newsprint that said, "WE LOVE YOU MIKE!" like something six-year-olds might make in art class to send to a classmate quarantined with the chickenpox, and hung it on the wall in front of his bed. At the time, Mike didn't seem to see it, or didn't acknowledge it, but later he would occasionally ask to have it moved this way or that to keep it in his line of sight. There were many things hanging on the wall in Mike's hospital room: his friends brought him cards, photographs of their children (these from the lesbians), stuffed toys, a picture cut out of a magazine of a grinning, brown-skinned man with no shirt on, just Mike's type. But Timo's sign was the only thing he seemed to take note of.

He confided in Jenifer, who would sit with him for hours in the evening and knit while he lay in bed half-conscious, grimacing and twitching. His eyes opened suddenly, and he whispered to her. She bent close to hear him. You had to put your head right next to his lips; he didn't have the strength anymore to project his voice. "I'm having an affair," he said. "Guess with who." She couldn't guess. "Timo. We sneak off when the nurses aren't looking. *Don't tell anyone.*" He closed his eyes and smiled peacefully. Awake, he asked his visitors reasonably for food, for drink. He kept us hopping. The secret was that he'd retreated completely into his dreams, leaving us with only the shell of his body to tend to, and there his life continued full of travel, beauty, and unexpected romance, as it had always been, only better.

During Mike's last five days, he stopped responding to anyone. Loie pleaded with him, "Stay with it. I'm right here. You can get through the pain." When she left, I said loudly in his ear, "Go! Go! It's okay to leave!" I had the nurse turn up the morphine. Mike wouldn't squeeze our hands. He didn't start at loud noises. His eyelids fluttered when the nurses changed his bed, and he wailed as they turned him this way and that. His face grew yellow and his cheeks hollow. He bit his lower lip, he groaned and writhed.

But that was just his body.

Too Nice

Mike was the opposite of materialist. In all realms of life, he made the most of whatever came to hand. He was the son of a mean, ignorant family, yet he developed himself into someone who was deeply contemplative, broadly experienced. And then, AIDS. All the characteristics that had been his—that he had worked to make inviolably and essentially and forever his—were his no longer. All his achievement went for nothing. His eccentricities were no longer simply his ways of doing things, his private pleasures. Instead, he required a widening circle of people to effect them.

No wonder he hated us.

He was so sick of being indulged. Privacy and the inner life—he could barely remember them. The privacy of AIDS is the privacy of intensive care, where the walls are curtainless windows, and there are no doors in the doorframes; it is the modesty of the hospital johnny, open in the back to expose the bum and too short to reliably cover the genitals.

I was giving Michael a ride to his Prison Book Project meeting one afternoon. I was turning left from Centre onto Seavern, we were almost there, and he began berating me.

"You're too nice," Mike sneered. "Not everyone is like that, but you are."

Too nice.

That was hardly my problem.

No doubt Mike had sensed the corruption that underlaid my attempts at generosity: the resentment, the jealousy.

I stopped myself from saying, nicely, "I'm sorry."

Neither did I say, "Fuck you. Get out and walk to your fucking meeting, then."

I drove on, I waited as he fumbled with the key to make sure he got into the building safely, I called him the next morning. He never mentioned my niceness again. Fran used to drive him home after the meetings every week, and she was neither too nice nor not nice enough. She was one of those other, better people—okay?

In the old days, Mike and I worked together. We respected each other, we enjoyed each other's company, we even loved each other, which may be hard to believe—but we couldn't anymore. We were no longer the people we once had been. Not since AIDS.

So why did I do it? Why did I try so hard to care for him? I don't know. How could I? I live in a post-Freudian society, and I don't know my own mind. I was trying to do good. But acts that appear benign may spring from malicious motives and have ravaging effects. Or, on the other hand, not. We may say these effects are unintended, but we can't know what we intend. Not without years of costly therapy.

I was overwhelmed, it was all too much for me, how could it not have been? I wanted to run away, I wanted it to be over. I'm sorry. I wish, I wish, I wish *every single day* that I had been more genuinely kind, more open and loving and freely generous. Although if it happened again, someone I know having AIDS—and it has, it will—I'd do it again and feel the same, because that's what AIDS does, the fucker.

Still, I think I helped him. I think things were easier for him because I was there—more so than if I hadn't been. I think I can say that.

Going Shopping

Michael used to shoplift. He didn't believe in spending money on food. He believed it should be free, everything should be free, and he was a man who acted on his beliefs. Like, food for the people, of whom he was one. At the Star Market within walking distance, the one on his corner, they caught him with cheese in his pocket. It wasn't the first time, either, and he was lucky he was too obviously sick for them to totally throw the book at him. They barred him for three months. Typical Mike, to place that kind of obstacle in his life for one of his wacko dogmas. Fuming, I drove him out to the Brookline Stop 'n' Shop, where he and his thieving ways were unknown.

The shopping cart of a PWA is full of Gatorade: the Official Drink of Persons With AIDS. Diarrhea, night sweats, they lose those electrolytes fast. Also, as a hedge against wasting, high calorie treats: Häagen-Dazs, the Official Ice Cream. Brown rice and tofu, because macro diets might turn out to be the miracle we've all been waiting for. Fruit's too much trouble, it has to be peeled, and it's hard to know when you've cooked the chicken enough or the eggs. Too bad, because the virus lowers cholesterol, little known fact, it's one thing you don't have to worry about. But even people with immune systems get salmonella.

Grocery shopping with Michael I was forever complimenting myself on my tact in concealing any feelings of embarrassment about being seen with someone who looked like him. His clothing was filthy and torn and his countenance gaunt and gray. He did not shave every day nor shower. There was no longer any flesh on his legs or arms, and the neuropathy in his feet caused him to reel and stumble. People looked at us, it wasn't just my imagination, and I wondered who they thought I was to him: Wife? Nurse? Social Worker? (Was I hoping they didn't realize I was simply his friend?) The overwhelmed elderly crept along in every aisle, asking if I would just read them the small print ingredients or lift something down from the top shelf. They trusted me with Michael by my side. They could see I was a nice girl. Michael ignored them — and me when I reached and read.

He didn't cook, although he was a grown man who liked to think he could take care of himself. He ate from cans and packages, slurping and shoveling hurriedly. He spoke oddly of food; he said he put it into himself. For example, he would say, "I *put in* two slices of toast and a hardboiled egg this morning." He said the same thing of his medications: "I *put in* two acyclovir and a megase." As though his body were a machine separate from himself, a slot machine, one that was fixed from the outset to prevent the exhausted gambler ever from winning a round. Or a receptacle: a piggy bank, a suitcase.

To me, who, unlike most of my generation, was nursed as a baby, to whom food is pleasure, sociability, a comforting suck, Michael's attitude was hateful. I'm *healthy*, though — that is, I don't have AIDS. That's the difference. Or one of them.

We shopped. He dawdled over every purchase and took me chasing around the store each week for the new, wonderful product someone had told him would be the ideal food: curative, delicious, easy to prepare. Non-dairy cheese. Lean Cuisine. Carob-flavored soy milk. The one food he consistently liked was Jello pudding. It came ready to eat in little plastic cups, and he preferred the tapioca.

He paid in cash, slowly counting out twenties from his wallet. I always worried he wouldn't have enough. I pay for my own groceries by check, but he obviously prepared for our expeditions by going to the bank. The new bills stuck together. Getting the bags up to his apartment worried me also: I fretted about finding a parking space in front of his building and about his insistence on lugging his share. I grabbed the heaviest bags before he could get at them, and I walked up the stairs behind him, to cushion his fall. I could just see him toppling backward onto me, sending us sprawling amid food and broken bottles on the hard marble floor of the bottom landing. Someone would have to rescue both of us.

Once we got the stuff up to his kitchen, I would leave. It was a small, grimy room, and I hated poking around, trying to figure out Michael's system. He never agreed with my placement of things. I would kiss him goodnight and run down the stairs.

Running felt good.

The Straight Yoga Class

Mike wanted to learn t'ai chi. Why not? The old folks in documentaries on China who move so gracefully under the trees in Beijing parks don't look any less frail than he did. He bought a book and cleared some space in his study, but somehow he never got anywhere with it. It was a project he was always meaning to do. He was interested in yoga too—I noticed a paperback next to his bed with a picture on the cover of a vigorous fellow looking supremely pleased with himself, practically ready to levitate, his legs twisted into a full lotus. Occasionally Mike tried a few *asana*s with an instructor who appeared on cable TV. So I invited him to my yoga class one evening.

He had lost a lot of muscle in his arms and legs, and he had never been particularly graceful, although strong and handy with tools. I told him to do only as much as felt comfortable and to relax on his back and breathe deeply if the class moved onto things that were too strenuous. During an exercise we were instructed to try in pairs, the teacher came over to help Mike and me. "I'm having trouble with this one," Mike explained to her. "I've been sick, and I have some neuropathy in my feet. It's hard to balance."

She had obviously never heard that word before. She didn't know what it meant or the particular illness it implied. It's true it's a long word, a medical word, but it had been part of my everyday vocabulary for years. I remembered how it sounded the first time—unpronounceable, slippery of meaning. The teacher was gentle and encouraging in suggesting alternative exercises, but it was obvious that she didn't speak our language, mine and Mike's. She'd never heard its nouns: *neuropathy, cytomegalovirus, mycobacterial avium intracellulare, Hickman catheter.* The AIDS language.

Mike and I didn't discuss the class afterward, and he never suggested trying it again, and I myself gradually stopped attending, although it was something I had been doing regularly for a long time.

Mike's Roommate

For years Mike had a roommate, John, but John stopped paying rent once Mike got sick, figuring no doubt that Mike could hardly force him to, just let him try. He wasn't so happy about having to live with a guy with the virus. They'd had sex a few times when John first moved in, but during most of the time they'd lived together they'd barely spoken, and Mike ended up with the little spare bedroom while John kept for himself the sunny parlor with the bay windows and wouldn't even have lifted the phone to call an ambulance if Mike had needed one.

Finally, after paying John's rent for four months, Mike kicked him out. Then he felt sorry for him and gave him yet more money to put toward a security deposit on a new apartment, essentially *bribing* him to leave, when, if there'd been anything of value in the place to steal John would've. I can just imagine him pocketing something on his way out the door, a handful of Mike's pills, maybe, to try and sell on the street, those were valuable as hell, not that anyone would have wanted them. I never said John was smart. Mike's pills cost about a thousand dollars a month, and the way Mike's lousy health insurance worked he had to front the money, then wait for the company to get around to reimbursing him. I and several others had taken up a collection because after Mike was discharged from the hospital he didn't have anything like a thousand dollars to pay for that first month of pills, and at his request I kept the money we raised in my bank account so as not to screw up his disability application. So I know that Mike used some of that money to pay off his roommate, although John had a perfectly good, steady job as a security guard. John had a lot more resources than Mike did, after twelve years at *GCN*, but Mike didn't see it that way, he saw John as an underclass waif of the streets who needed his help and guidance and who was entitled to be paid back by society, by Mike as its representative if no one more appropriate stepped in, for his deprivation. That was what had attracted Mike in the first place. He asked him to leave only with the greatest reluctance. It meant giving up a certain kind of opportunity.

Mike's Coat

Last night Roberta and I watched this show on public television that reminded me of Mike's coat.

It was a documentary about four elderly brothers who were dirt-poor farmers in upstate New York. One of them was accused of killing another by suffocating him with a pillow. The accused said he was coerced into signing a confession he didn't understand and that his brother had died in the night of heart failure. The brothers had lived together all their lives in a tiny, filthy house full of junk. They were pretty weird. The townspeople rallied around them, although before the trial they hadn't had much to do with them, and eventually they were acquitted.

I kept saying, "Where's Roger Wilkins?" because my theory is that Roger Wilkins is in all public television documentaries, and Roberta kept saying, "Those brothers look exactly like Mike" — especially the accused murderer. They didn't really, except that they all wore mesh baseball caps and had deep-set eyes and prominent noses. I'd thought of Mike, too. I think it was the dark eyes and the way the bills of the caps and the facial bone structure threw them into shadow. In many shots, the brothers looked cold, shivering in weighty old coats on overcast days. The coats were layered with dirt and clearly not as warm as they once had been.

Mike's coat was an old down one. It was blue, his favorite color, although that was hard to tell. It just looked dark, and it was shiny with grime at the cuffs and collar. Before he was hospitalized for the first time with TB, Mike used to like to walk everywhere, striding into the wind, hands shoved into pockets. Once, because the exterminator was coming, I had gone to his apartment to help him move things out of his drawers and his closet, and there was his coat. When I hung it up on its hanger, it felt heavy for a down coat: the big pockets were full of rocks, rubber bands, notepad, pens, and it was so old the down had lost its loft.

After Mike got out of the hospital, Jacoby took him shopping for a new coat. She was great at persuading him to buy things. She convinced him a new coat would be warmer, better. Since the hospital, he felt cold all the time. He chose a black jacket with a bright zip-out lining and patches of color here and there—red, purple. At first he was very proud of it and of himself and Jacoby for buying it. He told and retold the story of their shopping expedition. But, as with so many things, he eventually turned against the coat. It had stopped warming him. The zipper didn't work easily. He hated it. He castigated himself for being so foolish as to buy a new coat. But he didn't go back to the old one. He could have had it cleaned, but that wasn't the kind of thing he did, and he'd already violated one long-standing habit by buying himself the new coat, with poor results.

These winter days I often see Mike walking toward me on the sidewalk, a tall old man—his illness aged him—huddled into his coat, hands deep in his pockets, shoulders hunched, capped head drawn down to his chest against the cold. As we approach each other he looks up at me, and don't worry, it isn't him, not even close.

My Art, the Sea

Roberta and I rented a place in Provincetown for three months. It was during my teaching days, which fortunately for both me and my students are now over, so I had the summer off. Our plan was that I would live there and finish my novel, and Roberta would visit every weekend. The place we rented was a tiny cabin with a futon bed in a loft above the living room and the kitchen in an alcove that led out to a little screened porch, where I set up my computer every morning after breakfast. From the porch, you looked out into a forbidden garden. We were informed right from the start that it was for the use of our landladies only, who lived in the big house, of which our cabin had once been the garage, and ran a cute little store selling natural soaps, lotions, etc. It was quite successful with the summer crowd. I heard recently that they broke up, and it's all for sale — business, house, cabin. One of them used to wear a kind of shield of makeup that made her face look stiff and masklike, her eyes darting around behind it. The other was more down-to-earth, and she told me she wrote too — articles about her cats. I wasn't surprised to hear things didn't work out. They were nice enough to us once we completed our rental negotiations. Their place was clean and well-appointed, and they provided special soaps from their shop for the bathroom, one turquoise and one deep purple, to match the striped shower curtain. The soaps gave Roberta a rash when she used them on her weekend visits, but I liked them. We used only white soap at home.

Besides exiling us from their garden, our landladies wanted to forbid our having overnight guests, going so far as to write a special clause into our lease. I insisted on a compromise, and we finally agreed not to have more than two people staying in the cabin at a time. I was worried about explaining to Michael that I'd done something so bourgeois as to rent a summer home when I knew very well that most people are lucky to be able to rent even one home, and more fundamentally, I felt guilty about going away and abandoning him. I couldn't allow myself to get into a situation that would also get me off the hook as far as inviting him to visit. According to our lease, he would now be welcome only when Roberta wasn't there, which was just as well. She was much more likely to express her complaints about Michael overtly than I was. "Will he use the shower when he's up there?" she asked me, answering herself, "I doubt it."

But Mike thought my summer plans were great. He didn't mind the idea of Provincetown as I thought he would. Being from the Midwest, he had a thing about what he called "the Sea." He'd moved to Boston only after checking a map to make sure the city was on the ocean. Boston Harbor had turned out to be a disappointment, hardly the Sea, although he had discovered other natural features of the city, such as the Fenway, a swampy, desolate park where the gay men cruised in all weathers, that kept him there.

Roberta and I spent our first weekend at the cabin, very romantic, and then she left, and I called Mike.

He canceled the first visit we planned. He was feeling bad and had to see his doctor. That was perfect: I'd made a serious offer but had been relieved of the consequences. Every day I set up my computer on the little porch and stared out at the trees and the tomato plants, typing in a sentence or two once in a while, changing a word to a different word. My slowness at writing disgusted me. I'd been working on my novel for I won't even say how many years, but I couldn't speed myself up. At least in Provincetown I had the sun, the sky, no students, and none of their horrible compositions to grade. In the middle of the afternoon I packed a book, a towel, a bottle of water, and rode my bike to the beach.

I called Mike frequently — proving my dedication to his care — and we made a new plan once he was feeling better. I would pick him up at the bus station in Hyannis, because the connection to Provincetown is terrible. There are two different bus companies, and they refuse to synchronize their schedules. Then, typically, he insisted on going the whole distance by himself. He called me not from Hyannis but from down the street. I found him sitting on a bench looking too thin and pale and exhausted to have come to a resort. He let me take his bag, and we walked slowly down Commercial Street.

He wanted to buy a hat, a beach hat. He'd probably thought it out on the bus. Michael's clothing may have been old and ragged and dirty, but not out of lack of vanity—in fact, vanity was a sin for which he often criticized himself. He looked the way he wanted to look, at least until he got sick and began losing weight and getting skin eruptions. He usually wore a hat of some kind to hide his bald spot. When I first knew him, after his European years, he wore a Greek fisherman's cap or a black beret. Then he changed to baseball caps, the kind that are polyester mesh with an insignia in front and a plastic strap in back to adjust the size. For years he had a green and white one that said "Victory Garden," which I'd given him. It had been mailed to my attention at *Gay Community News* as a promotion for a local television show, and it gave Michael great pleasure, since he was not only a lover of flowers and all growing things, but also a nightly frequenter, as I've said, of the Fenway Victory Gardens. However, the Victory Garden hat was long gone, the plastic strap broken or whatever happens to those kinds of hats, and Mike, wearing the plain navy blue cap that had replaced it, imagined himself among the throngs of carefree guys in shorts wearing something jauntier.

"Sure," I said. "There's a store that sells nothing but hats right around the corner." I immediately realized I'd made a mistake. The store was bound to sell hats for exorbitant prices that Mike not only could not pay, but would object to on principle. He'd be outraged that I had taken him to such a place, and he'd hold it against me. I couldn't think of anywhere else to go, though, for a hat. There was nothing like Woolworth's or K-Mart. However, our shopping detour was amazingly successful. The store was displaying a pile of sale hats that included a straw fedora that fit Michael perfectly and gave him a whole new appearance, like he'd come from a different era, and I remembered that he was ten years older than me. He looked like one of those male movie stars of the forties and fifties who always wore hats, if they had also dressed in rags and been terribly sick.

He was very pleased with his hat, and the rest of the afternoon was easy. We shopped for dinner at the A&P, where Michael, relaxed and magnanimous, also bought a beach chair — which he insisted on leaving with me as a present and which I still take to the beach even though in my opinion it's very uncomfortable. Roberta says it's good for her back. In the evening, I cooked and Michael rested, and then we ate and talked on the little porch. I was a little distracted during our conversation because I was busy telling myself it was fine, fine, just fine having Michael to visit, and he fell asleep early.

I lay up in the loft reading *Madame Bovary,* which my friend Stephen, who was also writing in Provincetown that summer — rather more successfully, since his novels were getting finished and published — had told me was his favorite book in the world. Well, it's not mine. I thought of various things I wanted to do instead of read it, but they all involved climbing down from the loft and making noise around the cabin that would wake Mike, so I tried to turn my attention to the book. I fell asleep early, which I hate.

I was very rigid about writing for a prescribed amount of time every day, from 10:00 in the morning until at least 2:00 in the afternoon. After all, it was what I had come for. Mike understood my purpose and even endorsed it, although he hadn't seen what I was working on — hadn't asked to see it, actually. My novel was about *Gay Community News,* he knew that much, and I was sure he would find it superficial, not to mention distorted, even for a novel. I had those criticisms of it myself. Once I had shown him a piece of it in which he had a cameo, and he called me up very annoyed because his character called a cab. Never in his life had he called a cab! — that was in the days before he was sick. I tried to explain that a character in a book isn't exactly the same as you, walking down the street. My plot, such as it was, demanded that *someone* call a cab, and for various reasons it made sense for Mike, or rather, his character, to do it. Although had he been in such a situation in real life, which was not inconceivable, he would have stuck to his principle of non-cab-calling; he, or someone like him, would have found a way around it, so my fiction had sugared-over the true complexity of the situation.

Anyway, both Mike and I had imagined that during his visits I would be creating like mad in the little cabin while he communed with the Sea, encountering there lovely men similarly occupied. So we both had our plans, but they didn't work out.

We had forgotten that he was sick.

A sick person cannot simply decide to meander around town and beach by himself whenever and for however long he pleases. He lacks the healthy person's measure of strength and imperviousnessness to the sun and the heat. Nevertheless, Mike insisted that I drive him out to the beach and drop him off. We arranged a time and place where I'd pick him up later. He walked off laden with nothing more than the usual beach paraphernalia — sunscreen, sandwich, water, book, new hat, new chair — but I could see he was finding this almost more than he could manage. He set off slowly through the parking lot, and I drove home and sat in front of my computer and stared at the screen for the appointed length of time, accomplishing nothing, entering a comma, deleting it — like Flaubert, although, obviously, without Flaubert's genius.

Hours later, back at the beach parking lot, Michael got into my car looking horrible, absolutely fried. The inaccessible men in the dunes with their tanned pumped up bodies had infuriated him, and he had been able to find no shelter from the sun. I felt it was my fault, and he felt that way too. I had known inside myself that I shouldn't have let him go — although just try stopping Michael from doing something he wants to do. Also, I had my Art to think of.

Why Provincetown, anyway? Why couldn't I have stayed put in the city to write? Provincetown is full of light and flowers, and beautiful people dressed in silly, gorgeous clothes who go to tea dance every afternoon and out to dinner every night if they feel like it. They have summer romances, even their old relationships are summer romances. They shriek and kiss in the streets, lesbians too. I would hear their laughter ringing down the narrow alleys at night. Provincetown is the opposite of Mike, maybe of me too. He was never silly, never carefree, never on vacation.

The next day while I wrote, he visited an artist friend of his who he knew because when she used to live in the city she had been a GCN volunteer. She went off to work after a while, and he hung around her living room reading a book of poetry she had recommended to him by a friend of hers with AIDS. The walk back to my place from hers was too much for him, not that he called to ask for a ride or anything, and by the time we left for Boston—I was driving him back—he wasn't speaking to me. In the car, he half-lay beside me, the seat-back pushed down as far as it would go, totally silent. When we finally got to his apartment, I helped him out of the car and carried his luggage up the stairs. He didn't say goodbye. We never mentioned his visit to Provincetown again, nor the possibility of another, and for the rest of the summer I drove back to Boston once a week or so to see him.

Mike complained every time he had to get in or out of my car. The door on the passenger side needed oiling—still does—and it was hard for him to yank open or closed. Healthy passengers didn't notice it.

Memphis Stories

Going to Memphis

The beginning of the end: for me it will be one thing, for you something else, for Michael it was changing planes in Memphis, Tennessee. He collapsed in the airport, and the security guards took him to the nearest hospital. When he awoke, they were looming over him. How he hated the police.

Michael never intended to go to Memphis. He was on his way to Austin, Texas, to visit his old friend David. For ten days he would be someone else's headache, and I couldn't wait.

He had been collapsing even before he got on the plane — pitching right over, and he was tall, he was like a tree falling in the forest, and maybe he hadn't made a sound if no one was around to hear him, not even the most delicate ripple in the air to prove it had happened, so he didn't tell friends, doctor, anybody. He was paranoid that we would try to dislodge him from his apartment if we knew, and he was right. Like they used to say in the sixties, just because you're paranoid, it doesn't mean that they're not out to get you. I, for one, didn't approve of his living there all alone. It wasn't a safe place for a sick person: up three flights of stairs, and then once you were inside it was cluttered and dusty, a breeding ground for opportunistic infections.

But Michael loved his apartment in the Fenway, wouldn't consider for a minute a move that would take him out of the neighborhood. Not only was it the venue of his sexual success, but from his bedroom window he could see the tops of the trees that overhung the Muddy River. Stars, flowers, rocks, shells, animals hiding in the woods — these were important to him. In the packages he sent to prisoners he included *National Geographic*s and pages from old Sierra Club calendars; he believed they cherished, as he did, a glimpse of the outdoors.

I'd made a call without his knowledge to the AIDS Action Committee to find out if there weren't some kind of AIDS home with someone to cook his meals and take care of him in an emergency and an elevator instead of three longer and longer flights of stairs. There wasn't.

Until he got out of the hospital the first time, even Mike's closest friends had never seen his place or met his roommate. After that, we were allowed to visit. A brigade of lesbians came over and painted and moved the furniture around. Others of us cooked, cleaned, took him out on errands. But for the most part he tried to manage alone, and he claimed he liked it that way. I wonder, though. Shouldn't we have insisted more firmly? Medicaid would have given him a home health aide for twenty hours a week. My friend Walta got one, as well as a nurse, a hospice worker, and two buddies, not to mention a lover who watched over him twenty-four hours a day. Walta collapsed too, but someone was always there to catch him. At least someone should have come around to Mike's regularly enough to make sure he hadn't fallen in the bathroom and hit his head on the radiator. He had come to covered in shit.

"It was very strange," he admitted to me weeks later with a kind of scientific interest. "I was paralyzed. I couldn't move. So after a while I decided to go back to sleep, there on the floor. What else could I do?"

When he woke up again, he crawled to the phone and dialed the only number he could remember—Larry, who rushed over with his boyfriend in tow to do the mopping.

I was furious he hadn't called me. The brain is a funny thing—his and mine both.

"You see? This is how I live," Mike concluded bitterly. I didn't understand his point. Because we'd been talking about how he wouldn't tolerate a home health aide, a stranger in his apartment.

I assumed such a terrible thing could only have happened once or Mike would have told me about it, even though he didn't tell me about the Larry-incident until weeks after it happened and even though I knew for a fact that it had happened more than once, because I was with Michael when he collapsed only two days before he got on the plane. We had gone to the Monday night dinner for people with AIDS. I was always trying to persuade him to go, because they served a lot of food there, a lot of variety, contributed by various restaurants, and Mike had begun complaining that he was sick of everything he could make and everything anyone could make for him. The fact is, eating was not what it had been. Proper digestion was a thing of the past. Instead, he shat, he vomited. Still, if nothing else, I thought, and he eventually agreed, it would help him to meet other PWAs. All of us lesbians in his life, and Larry, we were nice enough, and not unfamiliar with the issues either, but I felt Mike needed to be around his fellow *suffarahs,* as they say in Jamaica. People with experience who would commiserate and advise.

Not that he was particularly friendly to anyone when we got there. And then a guy sat down to talk to us who had just moved in with a bunch of Buddhists. He began haranguing us about Buddhism, meditation, quality of life, and so on. It wasn't a very Buddhist thing to do, and it made it impossible for Michael and me to talk together without rudely ignoring him. So we ate in silence, avoiding the glittering eyes of the Buddhist, and then afterward I told Mike to wait for me while I ran to get the car. When I drove up, he was lying on the ground, and the other PWAs were crowded around him. I had told him to *sit* on the steps, but he had *stood* there waiting for me, and I had *run* to the car, but his legs buckled under him as soon as I was no longer there to catch him. He missed cracking his head.

So someone like me, or Larry, should have persuaded him that he was in no condition to fly. But I was looking forward to time without him, maybe his other friends were too, maybe even Larry, and he didn't tell his doctor about collapsing, so his doctor didn't find out it was because of his heart, his heart was failing, and he didn't tell him not to go, and anyway, who ever persuaded Michael of a damn thing? He said he was fine, and no one wanted to risk making him angry by questioning him—Michael was quite capable of holding a grudge. He was an adult with a ticket who wanted to see his friend David and warm, sunny, laid-back Austin, Texas.

At first Memphis seemed to be an annoying delay, but not a disaster. Mike called me just as I was going to bed. He said he was fine.

He didn't explain why he had ended up in the hospital—probably he wasn't sure. But he sounded strong and cheerful enough, laughing at himself and planning to move on in the morning.

So I didn't call him immediately when I woke up the next day, and I didn't even call as soon as I got to the office. I didn't call at my first opportunity. Between the time I woke up that morning and the time I dialed the hospital, I was calm. I should have known better than to have believed Michael, since he apparently felt that waking cold, filthy, and immobile next to the radiator was acceptable and in fact preferable to allowing a helper into his apartment, but I went to work, sat down at my desk, arranged a few files, made coffee, whatever, then I said, "I think I'll call Michael."

Only then did the emergency begin. For me, of course, not for Michael. The switchboard operator put me on hold because she couldn't locate him. He'd been moved from his room to Intensive Care. A nurse came on and said, "A cardiac event, a blip, a spike." His blood pressure had fallen, his lungs had filled with fluid. A sudden pneumonia or something. They were terrified that he would die on them and forced a respirator tube down his throat. She advised me to come right away, as soon as possible. Mike had dropped down upon them from the sky, dying of AIDS, and they wanted an explanation.

Early December: I wore my parka to the airport in Boston, and then it was warmish down South and drizzling. In Charlotte, North Carolina, I bought magazines and called the ICU from a payphone. Southern Bell: it wouldn't take my credit card, and I had to use change. The nurses, the doctors, the receptionist, they were all awaiting my arrival.

From the Memphis airport I took a taxi through flat land past condo developments and strip malls, one after the other, that was all there was to see. Elvis Presley's pink Cadillac was parked in the lot of one of the fast food places, his private plane in another. I stared out at blinking lights, red and green—Memphis was full of Christmas. (Mike would have written *xmas* there, as he did on the pad he wrote on while he was on the respirator, because of course he couldn't talk with the tube down his throat. He refused, on principle, to acknowledge the Lord and His Family whenever possible.) Every floor in the hospital was festooned with red and green bunting, more blinking lights, candy canes, little fake trees. The ICU nurses came to work wearing jolly Santa-head pins on their raincoats, with red eyes that lit up when you pulled a tiny cord. They said they would have come and picked me up at the airport. They felt just awful about the cab.

I asked them for the name of a motel, but they wouldn't hear of it. I was their guest. They would put me up in a room in the hospital, absolutely free. That's the difference between Memphis and Boston — they're so goddamn friendly down there, and the hospitals have long, disused corridors where they might as well put up visitors. There aren't enough sick people to go around in Memphis, Tennessee. They don't know from AIDS there, at least not in the big Methodist hospital out near Graceland and the airport.

So Mike and I were both in the hospital.

We were *hospital/ized.*

I stood at his bedside. I didn't think he'd be happy to see me. I thought he would be angry. Spending all that money, and for what? Just to be there. Later, he said, or rather, wrote on his clipboard, that my appearance amazed him; he hadn't known I was arriving — although he must have been told. He may have forgotten, or misunderstood, or thought he was having a dream. In the hospital it becomes hard to distinguish waking from dreams. First thing, I said, "Don't worry, my friend Ellen gave me her frequent flyer miles. The flight was totally free." The nurses were standing around us. They'd seen stranger relationships, there in the ICU. "I just pretended I was her at the airport. I made the reservation in her name."

He nodded. I sat down next to him on the bed and took his hand. "Oh, Michael," I said. He looked at me, he had big brown eyes, he shook his head, tried to smile. This wasn't his life. How could it be? All his work with the prisoners, their cruel and unusual punishment, the point was sharing his luck from outside. Surely this ordeal wasn't his to endure. Or anyone's. Now that I'd appeared, he would wake and find it had all been merely a dream. A *folie a deux,* perhaps, as it seemed to be my dream too.

The room was darkish, and he lay there, inhaling, exhaling, hooked up to the monitors recording the beating of his heart, the frequency of his breaths, and the pulsing of blood through his veins. The bed faced away from the monitor screens and the room's one window, which in any case looked out on a passage between buildings and to another window with an awning over it. Nothing interesting. In Memphis I sat on Mike's bed for hours facing him and the awning he never saw, watching as his heartbeat, his blood pressure, and his breathing speeded and slowed. Since the monitor screens were behind him, did he know they were there, or the window and the awning? I didn't think to tell him about them. To measure his blood oxygen level they taped a plastic clip to his finger, which he periodically tried to remove because it pinched, it bugged him. "Don't," I said, afraid a line on the screen would go flat, alarms would sound, and nurses and doctors would hurl toward us through the door, ready to break his ribs. Since he couldn't see the monitor, he couldn't know what the clip was for. A petty annoyance, to distract him from the major ones.

Maybe they put the monitors behind the bed deliberately. Maybe it's damaging to have the secret rhythms of your body constantly on display before you.

I try to remember the terrible sound of Michael breathing on the respirator, but I can't. The machine is a metal box on wheels, and just the other day I read that one of them blew up in the Bronx, and three patients were killed. The thing had been emitting sparks, but no one had paid much attention. It was in the *New York Times*. A technician wheels in the respirator, and twice a day after it's all hooked up, she returns to clear the tubes of saliva, mucous, and condensation. She puts on a mask and gloves and briefly detaches the tube from the machine and empties it into a bucket. She swabs the patient's mouth and throat, which are rubbed dry and raw from the tube's intrusion, and suctions out the fluids that have accumulated in his throat. I was angry that the technician didn't visit more often, and I pestered the nurses about when she was expected, because Mike's breath gurgled and there were crusty sores in the corners of his mouth. When she arrived, I was sent from the room. I could hear him gagging from the hallway.

That first night I got to sit with Mike only for about an hour. I held his hand and watched the monitors, trying to give him the full force of my attention, for whatever that was worth, trying not to become distracted or bored. It was what I had come for.

A nurse came in to give him his Ativan. She said he would soon fall asleep, and indeed his breathing and his heart rate slowed. The monitors confirmed that he was dozing off. She asked me to leave him alone while he slept and promised to call me in my room the minute "anything happened" during the night. She thought he was dying, but I didn't. I leaned over and whispered to him, "Good night, Michael. I'm staying in a room upstairs. I'm right here in Memphis with you. I love you." I kissed him on his high forehead. I didn't want to regret later not giving him a kiss, not telling him I loved him.

DNR I

Twice I talked with doctors about a DNR for Mike: Do Not Resuscitate, pull the plug, the Karen Ann Quinlan solution, and the second time it was real, life or death, or rather death one way or death another, but the first time, in Memphis, it was just doctors. They couldn't figure out what to do. Most people, we flail around for years on end unable to figure out what to do, but for doctors, it's their training, or maybe their heredity, they can't tolerate it like the rest of us.

I can sympathize, to a point—Mike drops down on them from the sky, his lungs filling with fluid, his heart rate slowing. "I have AIDS," he tells them, and whoa, they aren't ready for that at all, they send those cases to the public hospital downtown, they don't see that here in this godforsaken Methodist hospital out among the shopping malls. They panic, rush Mike to the ICU, and shove a tube down his throat. Then I drop down among them too, and *Jesus* are they glad to see me. Now they've got two alien visitors, but that's better than one. They can't figure out exactly how or why he belongs to me, but at least the guy belongs to someone.

They tell me the only diagnosis they know that goes with AIDS: PCP, that's the ticket. Never mind that the bronchoscopy came up clean. Diagnosis is an art. Later, in Boston when it happened again, the difficulty breathing, the collapse, the docs there knew right away: final stage AIDS, congestive heart failure. They saw it all the time. With gay men, HIV is like love, grabbing them first in the sexual organs, entering the lifeblood, lodging finally and irrevocably in the heart and the head.

On my second day in Memphis, the nurses shooed me out of Michael's room so he could sleep and then pulled me aside and asked me to wait until his doctor came in. He wanted to talk to me. They warned me not to be put off by the doctor's harsh, even brutish, manner. He's the best, they assured me, although he's not tactful, he doesn't seem kind, but he cares, oh he cares deeply about all of us, every single one, even some AIDS-ridden faggot.

They put me in a room with a bulletin board displaying mimeographed nurse schedules, some nurse magazines, a chair or two. No windows. A horrible, boring room. A room like a prison, like a Hell, and me waiting in it like the damned on the morning after a hellish day, airplane, ICU, Mike on respirator, practically dead.

After a while, I went down the hall to look for the doctor, but then I was afraid that he would arrive in the room, and I'd be at the other end of the hall, and he'd think I'd left. Which I had. I went back to the room, and then I got bored again and rushed out to the nurses' station, glancing around to make sure the doctor didn't slip into the room while my back was turned. He will come, said the nurses. We have faith.

And when he finally got there, with his famous straight-from-the-shoulder manner, what did he want? A DNR, from me. "Your friend is very sick," he began. I had brought my Health Care Proxy form with me, but now that I think about it, neither the doctor nor anyone else in Memphis ever looked at it. They just wanted a signature, any signature. "Tell him yourself," I said. You coward. He's conscious, he's lucid, he's got that clipboard and pen for writing down his thoughts. He's not even comatose. Crazy, maybe, but no more than he's ever been. You'll just have to deal. Clearly the doc wanted him out of the way. Not dead, exactly, but out of his hair.

"I'll discuss it with him," said the doctor. "But I'd like you to discuss it with him too."

Back in Mike's room I told him, "The doctor wants me to tell you you're very sick."

Mike gestured at the respirator. We looked at each other and rolled our eyes.

"I asked him to come in and explain to you himself what he wants."

Mike nodded and wrote on his clipboard: "I want to live." He signed and dated it.

"This statement is worthless," the doctor said angrily when I brought it to him. He was right — don't we all, or at least most of us? But Mike was right too; he still had some time left. Later, back in Boston, no, he didn't, it was a totally different story — but in Memphis he hadn't reached that stage yet. Not yet.

I saw a piece about exactly this problem in the *Boston Globe*. People with AIDS in hospitals where the doctors had little experience with it were encouraged to give up treatment because all the doctors knew about the disease was *Fatal! Fatal! Boing! Boing! Boing!* Might as well shoot yourself in the head. Fling yourself off a balcony. Do a fistful of pills. The reporter interviewed parents whose son had died, and others whose son had had the same problem in a different hospital, but who hadn't died. Or rather, who hadn't died at that point.

Anyway, Michael never signed a DNR. He always hoped that something would come along to save him.

Mike's Laundry

This is how friendly the people are in Memphis: the hospital Director of Social Services herself wanted to do Mike's laundry. She wanted to take it home and throw it in her own personal washer/dryer and bring it back sweet-smelling and pressed the next morning. The ICU secretary had directed me to her when I asked for directions to the closest laundromat. Neither woman wanted to tell me. The secretary claimed she knew of none. The director of Social Services admitted one existed, but she explained first that it was too far to walk and then that the neighborhood was too dangerous to walk in. But there were no neighbors. The hospital was surrounded by malls. I had a Krispy Kreme donut for breakfast and a Whopper for dinner, which are not the kinds of things I eat, ever, but I had to take what I could get, do like the Memphians do. That was why I went to look at the Christmas decorations at Graceland with the ICU secretary and her boyfriend. They invited me in a paroxysm of hospitality, and Mike, writing on his clipboard, urged me to go, but we never get out of the car, and I didn't see much, a few flickering lights. The estate is surrounded by a high brick wall.

There was a little bag in Mike's room containing the clothes he had been wearing when he collapsed. "I think I lost control of my bowels," he wrote to me on his pad. He was directing me in reorganizing his possessions, a pastime he enjoyed. I had occasionally done it for him at home also: following his instructions I'd clear off his night table or move boxes from one closet to another. I tucked certain items into his shirt pocket and arranged others on the rollaway table beside the bed: pen, memo pad, and checkbook in his shirt pocket; glasses, acyclovir, swabs, clipboard, bouquet of pink freesias (from me), and book beside the bed.

I hated the idea of Mike's soiled clothes stewing, forgotten, in a plastic bag in the overheated hospital room. He didn't want the bag thrown out—he was surprised that I suggested it, although what he needed these particular old clothes for I didn't know, since he had plenty of others at home, and even right there with him, in his suitcase.

So I told the director I needed to do a wash, and she offered to take it home for me. She was a smartly turned-out woman in a suit of Nancy Reagan red and a white blouse accessorized with one of those floppy, dress-for-success bows at the collar that no one up North bothers with anymore. I'm sure she was my age or even younger, but she looked so much more like an adult than I ever would—I really didn't want to burden her with Mike's shitty drawers. She didn't seem to have been informed of the specific illness from which he suffered.

We compromised. She drove me the three blocks to the laundromat, and I promised to call when I was ready for her to pick me up. It was raining out. In my opinion it's always raining in Memphis, although I didn't go outside much when I was there to verify this, and I have vowed never to go back. I bought a packet of detergent from the laundromat vending machine and shook Mike's clothes out of the bag into the washer without touching them. I berated myself alternately for being too fastidious and for not protecting myself with latex gloves.

It was a weekday afternoon, and the laundromat was oddly populated with fathers and children. The children zoomed around the machines and the fathers ignored them, talking together or watching soap operas on a big TV that hung from an armature bolted into the ceiling like the ones in the hospital. I sat in a green plastic chair in a row of chairs screwed to a metal rail and turned the pages of a tattered *People* magazine. When the clothes were done—hottest water, hottest dryer setting—I sniffed them. They smelled like soap. I folded them neatly in a stack which I tucked under my arm. I had thrown away the bag. One of the fathers directed me to a payphone, and soon the director came to whisk me away in her car. She couldn't have had much work to do.

The next week, after Mike had been taken off the respirator and moved to a medical floor, and I'd flown home, he called me to complain that one of the nurses had put him in restraints to prevent him from getting out of bed to use the toilet when she didn't answer his buzzer, because he'd fallen. I called the director, my old pal, to get them taken off, but she was no help at all. Finally, despite Mike's scorn for organized religion, the chaplain sprung him.

The Plane to Seattle

Sometimes Mike forgot he was in the ICU, and he thought he was on a plane. The plane to Seattle. "When do we get there?" he asked me. "How long have we been in the air?" Seattle—as far across the continent from Boston as you can go. He knew the flight was taking a long, long time.

I told him the story. "We're in the intensive care unit. We're in Memphis, Tennessee. You were going to visit David in Austin, but you collapsed in the airport changing planes. We're in Memphis, Tennessee."

He didn't believe it, but he said, "Oh, right," to humor me. He didn't know why I would lie to him, but I had the power, he didn't want to offend me. "Are we going home?" he asked carefully.

"Soon," I said. "When you're well enough to fly."

Ticket Money

As a kid I was fascinated by a book I found in the library about this retarded guy who is given a potion that makes him a genius—and then in his brilliance discovers that because of the drug his brain will eventually deteriorate past even his original feeblemindedness. It's written in the form of his diary as he watches his mind disintegrate, his character and penetration fail. It's a horrifying story.

Mike didn't rave in his last weeks; he was silent. He was struggling to hang onto himself, to keep his increasing confusion, memory loss, depression, hallucination in check so that to those around him it would seem like nothing more than his old, pre-AIDS eccentricity. He was struggling to remember his eccentricity. He said no one understood how hard his life was, and he was right. Some days people like me came over to help, but some days we didn't, and he had to remember to eat and drink and take pills, to nap and read *Leaves of Grass* and watch the yoga instructor on TV. To be who he was. Mike Riegle. Mike Riegle. Mike Riegle. Any kid knows how your name flies apart if you chant it over and over, the anomie, like spinning around and around and around on the playground until you can't see, you can't walk, you can't hear, you can't think, and you're ready to vomit.

He kept losing money. Mike Riegle cared nothing for money—but before he had always been careful with it. He knew it was necessary.

In Memphis, after they took him off the respirator, he was frantic to leave the hospital and to come home. Some deluded social worker at the clinic back in Boston told me Medicaid would pay to transport him in an *air ambulance,* and I became totally fixated on that as the thing that would save him, although I had no clear idea of what the *air ambulance* was. Other people would call me up wanting to discuss how to get Mike home, they'd been talking to him on the phone and of course he'd pleaded with them to get him out of there, and I would say, "Don't worry, the *air ambulance* is coming." I didn't want Mike to leave the hospital. I mean, I did, it was awful, since I left they weren't treating him well at all, but I was afraid another plane ride would kill him. And then, even if he survived the trip home, how would he live? He thought he could go back to living as he had been before Memphis, which wasn't great, but he'd been scraping by. But he couldn't. He was that much sicker. It was impossible. The social worker came up with ideas like the *air ambulance,* which as it turned out was not available after all because Mike wasn't sick enough, although it was hard to say how he could have been sicker, and after it fell through he stopped returning my phone calls.

Mike decided to leave anyway, without an escort and no matter what the doctors said about the risk of pneumonia in the pressurized cabin of the plane. He set it all up—my attempts to help, my faith in social workers worthless to him—he got himself a ride to the airport and everything, and then he couldn't find his cash to buy the ticket.

When he called me, frantic, we both assumed the money had been stolen—he hadn't put it in the hospital safe. I called the airline and charged his ticket to my credit card. Mike saved by Mastercard—so ironic, after the endless arguments we'd had at *Gay Community News* because as office manager he'd unilaterally canceled the collective's charge card agreement with the bank and thrown the stacks of triplicate forms and the little machine you process them with into the trash. They were elitist. He wanted nothing to do with them.

After he died, going through his things and cleaning out his apartment, Loie found three hundred dollars folded into his checkbook. The ticket money. Right where he'd put it. There were more bills stashed between the pages of various books.

While Mike was still in the ICU in Memphis, he asked me to get a refund for the part of his airplane ticket that he'd never used, from Memphis to Austin to Boston. I called the Northwest Airlines and followed their instructions, sending them the letters from the doctor and the hospital, the ticket stub—but they never responded. Mike never got his refund. Was collapsing in the airport not dramatic enough for them? Did they think they needed Mike's money? Why do I even think about the ticket, the money? Mike's dead. Northwest is no doubt going under like all the other airlines in this crashing economy.

My father used to drive us past Newark Airport, and as the planes rose over the Jersey Turnpike he'd point to them and say, "Impossible! Impossible!" Flying. I guess it is.

Mike Dies and Is Laid to Rest

DNR II

It isn't the moment of decision itself that is climactic, me and two doctors sitting crowded together at the end of a long, long table, like the guests at the Mad Hatter's tea party. They'd pulled me aside into a kind of classroom/storeroom, with a blackboard bolted to the wall and monitors of various kinds that were not being used at the moment shoved into a corner. They were reviewing for me the seriousness of Mike's situation, which any idiot could see, it was obvious, I didn't need two doctors to inform me of it. Mike's regular doctor, Richard, was on vacation. Peggy with her thick round glasses was filling in, nodding at the diagrams the resident who headed the ICU sketched on the blackboard as he explained to me in layperson's terms the deterioration of Mike's heart. The two of them looked at me anxiously to see if I was understanding them, if I was taking it all in.

"I'll sign," I interrupted, before they asked.

There wasn't much to decide at that point, and Mike and I both knew it would be that way, and so he chose me to do it. The only instruction he ever gave me, he said, or rather wrote, since he was on a respirator at the time:

"I want to live. It's the 'vegetable' question that I worry about."

Another day he whispered to Roberta, "I'm still a boy, you know." He wanted her to help him remove his hospital johnny and put on his pants, the garments of a human boy, because he was not yet a vegetable.

So that moment of choice is not the crucial moment, the central scene, the one that has to be written about or else. I don't have to write about it. Death before they pounded Mike's chest, broke his ribs, shoved the needles in his arms and the tube down his throat again—or during. My friend Berit, a former nurse, insists she's never known resuscitation to work. Betsy, her girlfriend—my ex-girlfriend, although that was years ago, she and Berit have celebrated a tenth anniversary, a fifteenth—also a former nurse, says that's not true, she still believes in it, but Berit insists. Of course, Berit's into her alternative, spiritual thing, she used to open the window in a room where a patient had died to let the spirit flee the hospital.

No, it's more the progress to that inevitable moment, and then after my conference with Peggy, Mike waking and refusing, now that he was once again available, to make any decision for himself. Peggy was sent in to explain it all over again, to tell him what she and the resident had told me. Mike's response? He warned everyone who came to visit him that she was trying to kill him. No one, myself included, ever admitted that Mike might be crazy, and it's true that his thought processes seemed to be what they had always been—he could be highly rational and intelligent, a genius, I really believe that, but also he often experienced serious lapses in judgment. Guilt. Paranoia. Obsession. Grandiosity. Satyrism. He never liked Peggy, and his visitors didn't either, but I did right from the start, because she explained things, and I trusted her uptight, schoolmarm looks, her round glasses like that character on the *Beverly Hillbillies* who the Clampetts hired because she knew how to behave properly no matter what the situation. Peggy was smart. She snuck Mike the question again like a needle slipped skillfully under the skin: "Would you accept treatment that would put you back in the ICU?"

She knew the answer to that one. He'd made it clear, ripping out his IVs and biting the nurse, threatening to kill himself and yelling my name so they called me in at three in the morning. I dressed and drove to the hospital, where the security guard had instructions to let me upstairs. I'd been there before at that hour, but with Mike in the car, lying terrified in the backseat moaning, "I feel strange, I feel like I'm going to die," and Roberta speeding on a short-cut to the emergency room that I would never have known to take, and I was so grateful she was taking us, because I would have gotten lost if it was just me and Mike, I'm always getting lost. His temperature was 94 degrees and falling.

"You mean *one-hundred*-and-four," said the ER nurse.

"No, I don't," I said.

By that last week, though, I knew the way to the hospital by heart, I knew millions of ways. I thought about Mike all the time, and I couldn't sleep or enjoy sex, food, work, companionship. Only in the hospital, looking at him, would my thoughts of him leave me. Sitting by his side was the only time I had a little peace.

It was a miracle to see him awake. He hadn't responded to anyone in days, and yet no one, visitors, nurses, Peggy, believed he was comatose; rather he seemed to be deliberately thwarting us. I've pondered this many times: our blame of him. We attributed such willfulness to him. His stubbornness was palpable. Or was it? Why didn't we conclude that his spirit was weakened and that he was doing all he could? No one imagined that he simply *couldn't* respond to us, try as he would, that he couldn't hear us, or that he could, but couldn't make his hand squeeze that of his visitor or force his eyelids to blink. No one discussed that possibility, because angry withdrawal was so completely his style. It didn't seem abnormal at all, in fact, you could think of his unresponsiveness as a hopeful sign, evidence that his character was intact.

The ICU nurse led me into his room and I took his hand. "Michael," I said, trying to sound gentle and calm, "I'm here. You'll die if you take out those IVs. This nurse is trying to help you." I actually believed that, too. I was terrified of what would happen to him if he pulled his IVs out—blood and medication spilling all over the floor. Mess and pain. They were giving him a great new wonder drug to regulate his heartbeat. They can only give this drug to you for two days, more than that will kill you—although if you need it, you're probably dying anyway.

With me next to him, Michael grew quiet. He was too sick. He couldn't fight them anymore. He'd sustained his anger as long as he could. We held hands and talked until he fell back to sleep.

Now, I realize that Mike was right. Yank out the IVs! Yell and scream! Do not go gentle! I understand this now. He wasn't getting better in the ICU. He was getting worse because, no matter where he was or what they did to him, he would get worse until worse was no longer possible.

The next day, Jenifer and I toured the AIDS hospice. The director showed us around: flowers, rugs, wallpaper. It was like a lovely country inn, except for the hospital beds in the guest rooms. At the end of the tour, the director sat us down in her office, and she was no longer the polite hostess.

"Look," she said, "we can cure his diarrhea. The hospital can't, but we can. We'll use things they won't. We've learned things here that they don't know. We've cured cases worse than his. I guarantee we can stop it within twelve hours."

I wanted to send him right over. I believed her, and I still do, I believe, but Jenifer was worried, would they give him acyclovir for his anal herpes, would they suction his lungs? And I was sure that Loie, whom Michael had made his alternative proxy, in case I couldn't for some reason perform, and whom I felt it was only right to consult, was against the whole idea, against our even looking at it, although she hadn't come out and said that. It seemed to me that she took the heroic approach. The hospice, stopping treatment, looked to her like giving in. Well, yeah, so? That was my feeling. It's Death we're talking about here. We all give in.

Fools! We were all such stupid fools! I have to include myself, because I didn't stand up for what I was thinking, although I had the power to. The legal power. But what's that worth? I've never liked wielding power, and I only see the necessity of it, the good of it, when it's too late, so Michael made a poor choice in me. I was the proxy—but I didn't want anyone saying I'd betrayed him, I'd killed him, afterward. That was a projection of my guilt and fear, I knew that even then, and Mike's friends spoke with the voice of Mike's own demented denial. They acted as though they believed what he told them: that the acyclovir was still working, that carob soy milk would cure him. They stocked the hospital refrigerator with it, and he sipped it through a straw or let visitors feed it to him with a plastic spoon.

Mike didn't want to check himself into the hospice. I knew that. And if I knew it, I didn't have the right to take him there anyway. Did I? Except that he'd set things up like this: He wouldn't answer my questions about whether he wanted to go to the hospice or Peggy's about whether he wanted to be resuscitated. He reiterated that he would never go back to the ICU. When the hospice intake worker Jenifer and I sent in to visit him asked, "Do you want Amy to decide?"

Michael nodded, "Yes."

The bastard.

He left it all to me. So, he didn't want to check himself in, but he wanted, maybe, to be checked in. By the time I figured that out it was too late. He didn't have the stamina to be moved. He stayed in the hospital, and he died there, although he had begged, many times, "Don't let me die in the hospital." He wanted to die at home, he said, and he well might have, if he'd fallen a few more times, or planned his ventricular arrhythmias better. But really he never admitted he was dying at all. "I want to live!" he wrote to me while he was on the respirator. His solution to the vegetable question. So he died in the hospital. In the end I fulfilled not one of his dying wishes, secret or open.

Rob said, when I was explaining the situation to Mike's friends that last week, when all of us, even Loie, had finally allowed that it might be time for the hospice, but when it was too late for that, "He really is dying, isn't he?"

Which proves that Rob's a blockhead. We were all blockheads, incapable of seeing what was manifestly before our eyes. Death. A dying man. His skin yellow, his face a skull, his eyes rolled back into his head. After Mike died four days later he looked no different, except that the terrible struggle of his breathing had ceased.

Roberta had been the only one brave enough to ask the nurse about Michael's diarrhea. "He isn't eating anything. What is it?"

The nurse hesitated. "The lining of his stomach," she said.

Sunday Morning

The nurses like to have one designated person to talk to, they don't like to be interrupted by phone calls from who knows who. I called the hospital at least twice a day, last thing at night and first thing in the morning, and in between I was there in person. If *anything happened* and I wasn't there, the nurses promised, promised they'd call me, so I should stop calling them all the time, but they never called me, any more than the mechanic calls to tell you what's wrong with the car and how much he's going to charge, so you can decide whether or not you want him to go ahead and fix it. You have to call him, you have to be persistent and annoying. He doesn't have to like you. I finally learned life's lesson: They don't have to like you.

There was an interval between the time I came home from the hospital in the afternoon and my next phone call to the nurses. That call was the hard one. Mornings I awoke to the situation in a panic: Mike had been dying while I slept. But during those late winter afternoons, the sky turning deep blue and deeper blue outside my window—blue, Mike's favorite color—I cherished the peace of ignorance about whether he was awake, asleep, breathing, eating, choking, raving, shitting, vomiting. When I'd been out of touch for a few blessed hours, the phone would start ringing—friends, wanting to know how Mike was doing, and I'd feel totally negligent. It was the only time they could reach me, because during the rest of the day I was either at the hospital or calling the hospital and tying up the phone. And they were sick of my machine: Beep. Hi! If you're calling about Mike, he's out of Intensive Care! He's been sleeping a lot, but I'm sure he'd *love* visitors! Beep beep. The message form is sanguine, a person can't absorb bad news from a machine.

Mike had been transferred out of Intensive Care because treatment did nothing anymore except drive him literally crazy with pain and immobilization. Screaming in the middle of the night, he had threatened that if they didn't release him from the ICU he would kill himself. Ha Ha. They moved him to a medical floor, but a few days later a hospital shrink appeared, all set to put Mike on Haldol—to "clarify his thinking," he said. "We have to take these threats seriously." For once, as his proxy, I was decisive. Permission denied. His thinking seemed clear enough to me.

I woke up around 5:30 on the Sunday morning after Mike had been out of Intensive Care for a week. I called the hospital—why not, they're there all the time, available to insomniacs. And the nurse said, "He's alert, he's talkative. Come over right away." There were two things she wanted me to ask Mike about: the morphine drip and the hospice. My last conversation with him.

The morphine shots weren't working. When you skin-pop it like they were doing it spreads through the body via the subcutaneous fat, but Mike didn't have any, so the drug just sat in a lump where they'd injected it. The nurses wanted permission to mainline it into his veins, but Mike and I had of course never discussed this kind of situation—whatever kind of situation this was. He hated rudeness, that is, people intruding on him, insisting on answers.

I suddenly realize he must have had total, idiot faith in my intuition. My feminine intuition, maybe that was why he liked us lesbians so much. Us girls' girls. He thought he wouldn't have to explain himself. He would simply be, and we would simply understand. In the old days at *GCN* he'd once gotten a letter from some nut, which was addressed: "Mike Riegle: Male Lesbian." Mike was tickled. He kept it, and he showed it to me and reminded me of it several times during that year before he died. Somehow, Mike contrived things so that even his nurses were dykes. (He did have one straight guy, who brought in his saxophone to play at Mike's sickbed. Gee, thanks, man.)

Mike had maintained his silence about the hospice also. Like Dorothy from Kansas, he told everyone he met that he wanted to go home. But that wasn't one of his options. He didn't acknowledge that. He wanted to take his treatments there, as he had done before, and die there, if it came to that, although he still, secretly, hoped maybe it wouldn't.

Mike had been withdrawing deeper and deeper into himself; his illness, his body, required more and more of his energies, required all of them. He was laboring, laboring. But on Sunday morning his struggle, for the last time, was suddenly, inexplicably eased. I entered his room, and he opened his eyes, he looked up at me, he smiled. There was a copy of *Leaves of Grass* at his bedside, a fat, attractive Penguin edition with a painting on the cover of old Walt in a straw hat and beard. His friend Barb had visited him the previous evening, and as she had read from it to him he had awakened. He was full of excitement about *Leaves of Grass* and Whitman. He told me the story of traveling to Washington to research Whitman's letters in the Library of Congress as a favor to Charlie, who had a grant that included money for an assistant. (Charlie is famous to this day among fundamentalists around the country for burning a Bible at a Boston gay pride rally. Legendarily promiscuous, unquestionably brilliant, Harvard-educated, Charlie always reminds you, when the Bible-burning incident is mentioned, that he burned his doctorate and his insurance policies along with the Bible, but no one remembers him for that. Why does he not appear in this narrative until now? He was Mike's closest friend, until Mike got really sick. Then he wasn't around much, although that was perhaps by their mutual agreement. Mike complained that Charlie's contrariness wearied him now that he was ill. Charlie visited in the hospital toward the end, massaging Mike's feet before going off to teach for a semester in Mexico, for which he'd gotten a Fulbright. I saw him at a party after he returned, after Mike's death, and he was proclaiming in his high-pitched drawl, "In Mexico, I am a sex goddess. At first I thought the boys were just being polite because I was a tourist, but they truly adore fat middle-aged men with big tits.") He and Mike had been interested in the letters Whitman wrote to a young fellow he met on the trolley, and after reading them, Mike recalled, he went out to some modern equivalent, in joyous emulation of his hero, and picked up the same.

Mike had instructions for me, a mission. In his apartment were his glasses, necessary for reading Whitman, and a bottle of acyclovir tablets, to cure his anal herpes. I remembered his first time in the hospital, when he had sent me over to his apartment to get something, and I was so *honored,* because he never let any of his friends, even Charlie, see his place. That was then. On Sunday morning I needed to talk with him, and here he was trying to send me away as though we had all the time in the world. We'd talk when I got back. On the one hand I wanted to follow his lead—chat about literature, buzz over to the apartment—but on the other I had my questions, and maybe he sensed that and decided to occupy me with a fool's errand. Because even though his request to me might sound reasonable enough, it wasn't. It's true he owned a pair of prescription reading glasses, but in real life he had rarely worn them. And at the same time that he was begging me to retrieve his acyclovir, the stuff was dripping directly into his arm by the bagful. I tried to point that out, but he didn't believe me, although why would I have been lying? That's our relationship right there: he put his life in my hands, yet he mistrusted even a straightforward statement of fact. The acyclovir is in the IV. No, he needed the pills. He was in great pain. If they were, in fact, giving it to him IV it wasn't doing any good. Only his pills would work.

"Michael, I'm afraid neither one will work at this point," I said. "The nurse says if she starts the morphine intravenously it may help with the pain."

"Yeah, yeah, yeah, okay, okay, okay," he said offhandedly, to get me off his back. He had developed an enormous capacity in his illness to focus his attention elsewhere, away from you. Of course, we both believed we were dealing with life and death issues: Whitman, morphine, acyclovir, hospice.

I agreed to go to the apartment.

Quick, quick, I retrieved the pills and the glasses, which were right next to the bed, where Mike said they would be. Next to them was a small beaded medicine bag that Mike's prisoner friend Bobbie Lee had recently made for him.

It now sits on my desk. It's red, with blue and yellow beadwork around the edges of the flap that closes it. In the middle of the flap is a compass design: a ring of brown beads and inside it a cross, each spoke a different color. Red points north; yellow, east; white, south;

black, west. There is one skyblue bead in the center. Inside the bag is a braid of sweetgrass, a rock, three squares of cloth — red, yellow, and black — and a tiny sac of herbs.

In healthier times a few weeks previous, Mike had read aloud to his visitors the letter Bobbie sent with the gift, describing how he had obtained the red fabric and created contraband sewing implements while locked up in maximum security. For over ten years, Mike and Bobbie had exchanged letters, photographs, and gifts. Now, they would never meet. Mike always wore another bag that Bobbie had made for him, a small leather pouch, around his neck and a beaded bracelet from him on his wrist, and we kept these things with him after he died. They were burned and scattered over the earth with his ashes. I took the new bag to give him, to pull him out of the madness of the cure of glasses and pills.

But when I got back he refused to take any notice of it. No time for friendship or the spiritual realm. Whitman also forgotten, he put on the glasses and stared intently for many minutes at the label on the brown plastic pill bottle.

"Would you like me to read it to you?" I asked loudly. "Do you want to try to take one? I'll get some water."

He ignored me, staring and staring. Who knows what he saw.

"That's the acyclovir that you asked for," I said. "I also brought the new medicine bag that Bobbie Lee made for you. Look!"

I waved it in front of his face, but he refused to move his attention away from the bottle. Like the grand old protest song, We shall not, we shall not be moved, naturally one of his favorites, belting it out as they dragged him away in cuffs. We shall not be moved.

After a long time he lay his head down on his pillow, and I took the glasses from his face and held his hand. He fell into a kind of sleep, neither refreshing nor dreamless, from which he awoke only to his death five days later.

Mike Dies Peacefully

In my memory, in my writing, I circle around it like a hawk riding a thermal. I close in upon it, but unlike the hawk, I never plunge. The moment of death. Here it is.

Friday evening. I'd been at the hospital all afternoon, and Roberta and I were going out to dinner. Our coats were on. One of us had her hand upon the doorknob, about to turn it, and the phone rang. "I'll get it," I said, out of habit, not because I thought it might be the ultimate call. I was going out to dinner. I wasn't thinking about death. Or, rather, I knew it was close, that it could happen any second, but I wasn't thinking that it might be *now* or *now* or *now*—this second.

"His breathing had been getting more and more difficult," said Rob. "He was really straining. But then, about ten minutes before it happened, his breathing eased. People were here, around the bed. He opened his eyes and looked at us, he sighed. And that was the end. We waited, but he didn't breathe in again. Michael died peacefully, Amy, I want you to know that."

Peacefully. If you want to believe that, go ahead.

"The hospital wants to know what to do with him," Rob went on. "Can you come down here?"

And that was it. Over. I hung up the phone. I waited to see if I would cry.

How do I feel? I asked myself. Kind of hollow.

Angry, as usual. Angry at Rob for saying "peacefully." Angry at the hospital for needing my signature on their forms. Angry at AIDS for intruding on our normal little lives and relationships and Friday night dinners and inflating them to this grand, tragic scale until they burst with pain and death. Angry at Mike for suffering and dying.

Here's what I'm thinking: What if there were no AIDS? It never happened. Mike never got sick. We might have had a falling out by now. I might never see him. Or maybe I'd call him every few months and give him dinner. I would never have been inside his apartment. Mike would merely be my friend, my old, difficult friend. I wouldn't think of him every day, as I do now, still. I wouldn't carry him around like a flame I dare not let gutter. He wouldn't approve of the way I'm living these days: going to work, going to the gym, going home. Not very political. Roberta and I bought an apartment in Provincetown. He would hate that. He wouldn't like this writing I'm doing about him.

Since the moment he died, I've taken him with me everywhere.

I didn't cry for him at all then, although I do now from time to time. I turned away from the phone, and Roberta took me in her arms. We hugged through our winter coats. "Mike is dead," I said. "We have to go to the hospital."

We went out the open door of the apartment. In the car I said, "Rob says he died peacefully." We looked at each other. I didn't have to say anything else. She squeezed my hand and started the car.

At the hospital they asked if I wanted some time alone with him, and I was curious, and also I felt from the way they said it that it was something I should want, so I went into the room. I'd never been alone with a dead body before. Mike—a dead body. He lay on his back, his arms outside of the covers. I saw the medicine bag around his neck. I didn't touch him, didn't want to feel him stiff or cold. I didn't talk to him, even in my mind. No point, he was dead. I didn't pray. I didn't know what to do, sitting there with him, so I left. Later, various friends of Mike whom Rob had called began arriving at the hospital, and some of them went into the room with the body and stayed for a long time, but I waited in the corridor and never saw Mike, corporeally, again. Eventually people from the funeral home wheeled him away. I'd given a nurse the name of one that didn't mind burying people with AIDS. Roberta remembered it from the obituaries.

The nurse let us gather in the solarium at the end of the hall. All week I'd had conversations with doctors in this room, sitting in big vinyl reclining armchairs, the kind in which they seat patients recovering from surgery. No hope. Nothing to be done. We can make him comfortable. (Their irrepressible confidence, the optimism of power. Would they, too, describe Mike's death as "peaceful"? Maybe as "comfortable.") It was night, and the lights of Boston twinkled below the hospital tower. We stayed around to comfort each other, but Mike had kept his friends unknown to one another, and even after everything we'd been through with him and each other, we remained separate, it was hard to comfort. Not many were crying, although some probably went home later and cried. We ordered pizza. We sat in a circle and told our stories about Mike. We tried our best. Finally, we'd stayed long enough, and it was okay to go home.

Leaving, I stopped to thank Mike's nurse. I hugged her. Suddenly I loved her and didn't want to let her go.

Obituary

(from *Gay Community News,* January 1992)

Michael Riegle, gay liberationist, prison rights activist, and longtime resident of the Fenway, died on Friday evening, January 10, 1992, at Beth Israel Hospital in Boston after a long struggle with AIDS. He was surrounded by friends.

Mike was born in 1943 in Gary, Indiana. His father was a steel-mill worker, and Mike, too, worked in the steelmills to put himself through Knox College, where he received his BA. His early love of poetry — especially that of Robert Frost, much of which he memorized — developed into an interest in the psychology of language, the subject in which he received his doctorate from the University of Minnesota. After receiving his degree, he taught college for several years at Franklin and Marshall College and then at Cornell. He spent most of the 1970s living in Europe, primarily Italy and France, where he worked as a translator, English instructor, and children's tutor.

Mike was an avid linguist, fluent in Italian and French. He also studied Russian, Spanish, Greek, and American Sign Language. During this past year, as his illness progressed to the point where he could no longer be as active as he once was, he began watching Spanish soap operas and Italian soccer matches on cable television to keep up his language skills. And he searched the stores to find a children's book on American Sign Language when he discovered that the young niece of a friend had a deaf neighbor. Communication was crucial to Mike, and he expressed this value in everything he did, from his political work to ensure that prisoners were not isolated from the rest of the world but were able to interact with those of us out in what he called "minimum security," to the intense, one-to-one conversations that he enjoyed with his friends.

When Mike moved to Boston in 1978, he threw himself into the local gay political scene. His involvement with *FagRag*, an anarchist paper with an emphasis on sex and politics, helped him develop his ideas on these topics, and Mike worked tirelessly to put out the paper with little money and an ever-dwindling collective devastated by AIDS.

After volunteering at *Gay Community News* for six months, Mike joined the staff in the beginning of 1979 as office manager, a position he held until last winter. During his years at *GCN*, Mike expanded the paper's policy of providing free pen-pal ads for prisoners into a unique program that provided lesbians and gay men behind bars with information packets on subjects ranging from safer sex and living with AIDS, to legal issues, to exercises that can be done in a jail cell; advocated for prisoners who were being harassed, denied medical treatment, or isolated; and regularly published writing by and about prisoners in *GCN*. As a result of his work with the *GCN* prison project, Mike became involved with other prisoner advocacy groups. He was a moving force behind the Redbook Prison Book Program for many years and also advised the American Friends Service Committee and the AIDS Action Committee about the concerns of prisoners. Over the years, Mike carried on correspondence with hundreds of prisoners, many of whom came to regard him as a close friend. Some of them affectionately called him "Mother Mike."

To the very end of his life Mike brought to everything he did — whether it was sex, gardening, singing choral music, reading, or stargazing — a sophisticated and original mind, a curious imagination, and a deeply rooted integrity. As weakened as he was by AIDS in his last year he continued his prisoner advocacy work and began editing a collection of letters from lesbian and gay prisoners. When he found himself no longer able to enjoy old pleasures such as cruising the Fenway he developed new interests. *King Lear,* which he reread yearly on his birthday, provided him with a powerful negative example of what happens to a man unable to change and with the inspiration to continue exploring the world and the people around him. He loved children, perhaps because they embodied these values of growth and exploration, and in addition to enjoying the opportunities to do childcare that came his way, he maintained long-term relationships with the sons of his friend Mary Toleno.

Everyone who met Mike was struck with his unique style of conversation, with the slow and careful way that he developed his ideas. Although his deep, gentle voice is now still, we continue to feel its reverberations.

> Years ago I recognized my kinship with all living things,
> and I made up my mind that I was not one whit better
> than the meanest of the earth. I said then, I say now,
> that while there is a lower class, I am in it; while there is
> a criminal element, I am of it; while there is a soul in
> prison I am not free.
>
> — Eugene V. Debs

The Great Blue Heron

I wanted nothing to do with a memorial service. My philosophy was that when Mike died my responsibility ended, and you know what? I used to think about that when he was alive. I dreamed of the day when I would have no contact with Mike's remains, his possessions, or his associates. Of course it didn't happen that way. I ended up with the ashes. In ashes begin more responsibilities.

They were heavy. A man wearing a black suit handed them to me in a shopping bag with a chic black-and-white lily motif. It looked like the bag from an expensive department store, if you could only place that lily logo. You could take a nice bag like that anywhere if you had to, or wanted to, and none would be the wiser. I had been sitting in a sort of waiting room, like an orthodontist's but plush, hushed, elegant — wainscotting, oriental carpets, empty crystal vases on the mantlepiece. Beyond the waiting room I could see into a small chapel. It was exactly the kind of place Mike hated — bourgeois, religious, its only purpose to conceal decay and corruption. His decay and corruption.

While I waited, I imagined that the ashes had been misplaced, discarded, improperly prepared. I would have hysterics in front of the guy in the suit and haul him into court. "There will be pieces of bone," Roberta had warned me. I knew that, okay? It's the thing everyone remarks on, you read it in books: "Oh my God, pieces of his bones!" Pieces of bone wouldn't surprise me at all.

Mike's ashes were in a perfectly cubical white cardboard box placed in the center of the lily bag. "If you plan to do anything legal, like interring them, the documents you'll need are in the box," said the man in the black suit. "Of course, you may do what you like — just be discreet." Then he *winked* at me, the moron. A little undertaker good cheer. I was furious. I had done everything, everything, and now I would obviously have to open the box and remove the documents. I had planned not to open the box. When I rose from my chair, the twisted paper handles of the bag cut across my palm, and its heaviness unbalanced me. Not too much, it wasn't unbearable, not at all, but I was sick of it, sick of yet one more never-ending thing. This was immortality, the afterlife — a box and then who knows what after that, but something, no doubt. The undertaker gallantly escorted me out. He held open the brownstone's beautiful carved wooden door, and a cold wind assaulted us, blowing sleet into our faces. I ran across the icy street to the car as the traffic light changed from yellow to red, the bag knocking against the back of my knee, almost buckling it.

The Monday science pages tell of strange dark stars in which matter is so concentrated that a small cube of it would weigh more than a refrigerator. More than our entire planet, actually. In fairy tales, weights that for the wicked are immovable, for the good are as light as dust.

Michael's emaciated body. The heavy, heavy ashes.

How did the box get to the memorial service? Jacoby and her girlfriend gave me a ride — normally Roberta and I would have gone together, but the day of Mike's service was also the day after her father broke his hip, and she had left for the hospital in Yonkers. He died four months later. As I stuffed myself into Jacoby's backseat wearing winter coat, hat, gloves, long underwear, boots — because the service was outside in the middle of January, after all it wouldn't have been appropriate to hold a memorial for Mike that was comfortable or easy to get to — I must have dragged behind me the lily bag and in it the box. I must have held it on my lap in the backseat as we drove and carried it down the street to the site on a path through the Fenway reeds.

Because I had the box, the memorial service could start only upon my arrival. In the lily bag I had brought *Leaves of Grass* — the last book Michael read — and a clamshell to scoop the ashes with — something natural, from the Sea, as he would have wanted. At the appropriate moment I read a few lines, and I took the clamshell and plunged it into the box. I flung ashes onto the path where we, the survivors, and at night, intrepid gay men, ready for a tryst no matter what the season, would tread on them. I didn't fling the ashes into the path on purpose, but they didn't scatter as far as I thought they would. So next, I grabbed a fistful. It wasn't so bad. We Jews wash our hands before reentering a home after a funeral anyway, to mark the separation between death and life and to cleanse ourselves of death. But also because we shovel. The mourners have to dig until the grave is filled, and it's a dirty job. This time the ashes rained, bones and all, into the reeds. I invited the others to follow me, but there was a moment of hesitation. The *goyim* didn't want to get near the box. Finally, knowing it was their duty to participate — after all, they organized the thing, not me — they took their turns. Some stood where I had, and some took a short walk away from the group. Some used the shell and others their bare hands. On the way back to the car I threw the lily bag and the box into a municipal litter basket.

A group of us left the memorial service together — me, Jacoby and her girlfriend, Loie, Jenifer, Larry, Rob, Fran, Stephanie, Carrie in her wheelchair — and Loie cried out, Look! and we turned around to look, and lo, making his way among the reeds and the ashes, in the middle of the city, was a Great Blue Heron. This is what I remember. The heron is a lean, long-legged, deep-voiced bird. He seeks his simple food alone. He is blue like a shadow. Loie cried out again: It is Mike's spirit! It is his totem!

I wish more than anything I believed that. The Great Blue Heron.

The Afterlife

Calling the Names

These days—these days in the Age of AIDS is what I mean—whenever we get together in large groups—gay pride marches, conferences—we call the names. Occasionally the list is prepared in advance, and celebrities read it from the stage. But more often it's a grassroots, participatory kind of thing, with those in the audience speaking as they feel moved. Sometimes I get into it and recite a few of the names I carry around: Mike Riegle. Bob Andrews. Tim Grant. Walta Borawski. Gregory Howe. Siong Huat Chua. Raymond Hopkins. In no particular order.

Then I wonder: why did I do that? What can it mean to these strangers around me to hear these syllables? They'll never know the whole story. But as the calling of the names continues, it becomes a kind of theater or living work of art—a tableau vivant, *perhaps, as in the old novels my dead friends and I used to love to discuss at our dinner parties or over the phone. The accretion of names reveals an image: a glimpsed freeze-frame of our lives hollowed out by loss.*

Until the names start to overlap and bounce off each other. The tableau breaks up. The audience fidgets. You can't see all that much of this AIDS devastation in a freeze-frame—it's more like, oh, a big, messy old slushball, and everything it rolls over adheres and becomes part of its cold substance. Will this calling of the names never end? It could, in fact, go on for days—although the MC halts it after a while. There is other business to attend to. We have not gathered only to call out names. Must we not make peace? Must we not move on?

But my teeth are chattering, my body humming. I can't stop feeling the reverberations. . . .

Ice Chips

I've taken a two-week vacation from work, which wasn't easy. No one else on the staff ever seems to take vacations, so I've developed a reputation for laziness and unreliability, which is pretty ironic and undeserved since I put in, uncomplaining most of the time, the same fifty- or sixty-hour week at the shelter as everyone else, doing what needs to be done—emptying trash, swabbing toilets, boiling up giant pots of potatoes, taking a woman who's on the verge of alcoholic seizures to the emergency room, coming back to the office to meet with the graphic designer at 6:00 PM since he won't answer his phone or his doorbell before noon, writing last-minute fund-raising appeals.

Michael would have approved of my job, and that helps me stay with it, because he was always so sure of what one should do, of right and wrong. He disapproved when I quit teaching, which caught me off-guard, since he considered college so elitist that most of the time he wouldn't admit he had gone, but on the other hand youth, working with them, setting up around them their first counterhegemonic adumbrations, could be seen as a good thing. No doubt he was envious, too, class after class of pumped-up young men, the babyfat barely worn off their bones, lounging in their chairs, staring blankly at the instructor, blinking "amuse me." I saw them differently than he would have, of course. They were a hulking part of the reason I quit. Their withering disdain. Their refusal to learn anything from women. And the girls were just as bad. They had a particular way of wearing their hair, bleached out and curled away from their faces, so that it took months before I could tell them apart. Jennifer? Kristy? Marie?

The whole time Mike was sick I was going on job interviews. I went to my second at the shelter on the evening I got back from Memphis, and they offered me the job the day before he died, their indecision taking roughly the same length of time as his crisis. So he never knew about my job, although I told him about it. I pretended that his spirit—although he was not yet dead, so it had not escaped his wretched body—was watching over me, influencing the collective process. After it was all over, when I ran into his friends and told them what I had been doing since, I would say, "Don't you think Mike would have approved?" He was never big on vacations.

Roberta wants me to take my vacation with her, but I can't, not if I want to be a writer. She's planning a trip to Paris, but I've saved my precious weeks to write. Middle of February. Snow everywhere, especially in the hills of western Massachusetts. I'm not staying at one of those mansions where they wine you and dine you and leave your lunch outside your door on a tray so you won't be distracted in the midst of an act of creation. It's more like a bunch of college students trying to save on the rent. A dilapidated old farmhouse with a rumbling, ineffective furnace, a sink full of dishes, shelves of dusty little plastic bags holding the gray powder of what used to be herbs— marjoram, cream of tartar—a sticky squeeze-bottle of Dr. Bronner's peppermint soap in the shower. And cats. Which really burns me up. I'm allergic. You'd think they would have said something about them in the brochure. The animals alone are enough to make me want to get right back in the car.

These are all excuses. The truth is, I'm homesick. I don't travel well—not that I've come that far to get to this place, and it's all of a half an hour outside of the town where I went to graduate school. I lived in this same area for four not unhappy years. In the middle of it Bob got sick, and I started driving to Boston every Wednesday to visit him. So I can't say life was totally blissful, either. Still, I thought I might enjoy coming back to the area's familiar natural beauty. Now that I'm here, though, I can't settle in, although they've given me, for no apparent reason, the nicest room—large, sunny, views.

I try to make the place feel like my own. I move the desk from the front window, where it looked out upon a never-used dirt road, to the side window, where I gaze upon untracked, snowy fields and distant hills. A cardinal alights in a tree, then flutters away. Now, that's an improvement. From my desk at home all I see is the brown triple-decker house next door, with its blistering paint and cracked windows. My window frames around it a rectangle of sky and the top of a big tree. A plastic bag has been stuck in the branches for a year, obscured in the spring and summer by leaves, reappearing late in the fall.

I set up my computer and printer, I arrange my books on a shelf. I brought a radio, and I plug it in, but then I'm afraid to turn it on, because it may disturb someone who is writing. One of the real writers. I sit down on the bed. I try to anchor myself, to remember that I've looked forward for months to coming to this place, but it's no use. I'm unhinged, free floating. I should be writing now, shouldn't I? But how can I? Who am I? I pull on boots and coat. The room came with a map of a walk one can take.

There's a woman who lives in the house all the time, a caretaker, and she goes shopping and comes back with an amazing number of bananas and eggplants and onions, and I can't think what we'll do with these ingredients. She doesn't like the idea of meat, but we guests ask her to get a chicken next time. Dinner is a group-made pasta thing. I chop onions and meet the other residents. There are only four of us at this time of year, three in the house and one in a cabin hidden in the woods. He's a cross-country skier training for a race. He tells us how he cut a track in the snow from the cabin to the house so he can ski over to use the bathroom. He writes too, he's starting a novel. By the end of his two weeks he plans to have 50 pages, and already today, he arrived, he skied 10 miles, he wrote 1500 words. They all produce quantities of words, both around the convivial table and then later at their desks, even the fellow with the room next to mine, a sweet guy. We have a mutual acquaintance in New York, and coincidentally I've brought her new book along. We both read it and agree it's astoundingly bad, although we still like her personally. He isn't even a writer. He's a musician who had the idea to write a play on a manual typewriter, and he's tapping away steadily whenever I sit down at my desk, like an all-day rainstorm, like a pianist practicing scales over and over and over and over.

But it isn't raining. It's silently snowing, shrouding the view. Leaning over the silent keys on my computer, I stare out the window. The skier moves across the field, and a squirrel skitters up the tree.

I call Roberta and tell her it's not what I thought it would be at all, the cats, I'm not inspired. I want to come home.

"Don't," she says. "Not after only a day. You'd hate yourself for it."

"It's like having to live with the people in my writing workshop," I quip. I call up a few other friends back in the city to tell them my joke.

I'm here to write about Mike, and all the books I've set out on the shelf in my room are about people dying. In one, the author describes how she cared for her mother who was sick with cancer: "bathing her, washing her hair, rubbing her body with fine French creams, feeding her ice chips, stroking her hair, her hands, and her forehead." She describes her mother's hands, how they remained beautiful throughout her dying. How she held her mother's hand. I read this list of loving, compassionate acts, and tears fill my eyes. She describes in detail the process of changing the IV, of holding a basin while her mother vomits, and of vomiting herself as she empties it. She is as factual as a scientist; she is, as it happens, a scientist.

Oh, why couldn't I simply love Mike and be generous!

Even when I did those same things for him, it was as though I hadn't. Because of the bad spirit in which I did them. By the time he needed to be fed ice chips, I was too angry, too confused. He was choking on them, for some reason everything he swallowed had started going into his lungs, but he loved them and even more the popsicles that we crushed up in a dixie cup and fed him with a plastic spoon.

Best of all, he loved to drink soy milk. He had become convinced that his diarrhea was caused by lactose intolerance. It was Rob who had suggested this to him and I blamed Rob, unfairly, because he had merely told Mike that he, like many adults, was allergic to regular milk and that his solution was to drink soy milk instead. Mike decided he, too, would drink soy milk and be healed. I thought Rob and the others were fools for pandering to these delusions. Not that I didn't pander myself. I fed Mike soy milk, I fed him ice chips, but in anger and resentment at his stubbornness, his refusal to do anything that would really help him, like go to the hospice. Instead, weeks of suffering in the hospital, madness in the ICU. He wouldn't talk with me about anything useful, such as the point at which he would accept a morphine drip, instead he begged for soy milk. Carob flavored.

But why is that so terrible? We all have our delusions, and soy milk was a small pleasure to him, more than that, a glimmer of peace and hope. But I hated every minute of feeding it to him, not because I hated feeding him—although I did, a grown man, it was too sad and pathetic—but because it was the food of his delusion. It was no use being scientific at the bedside of someone like that.

I never cried for Mike, but I'm crying now. I cry because I miss him, because I loved him, because I feel so mean, because his death was so terrible, hard, and early, and I didn't treat him tenderly, because my job is not working out and he would have wanted it to, because I'm unhappy in this place full of strangers and cats, because never in my whole life have I done even one thing right. This is why I hate to cry. All misery, great and petty, past and present, conflating in tears.

Influences from Beyond the Grave

Here I am, naked and sweaty in bed with Roberta, who I've known only forever but we've definitely never done this before, and suddenly Bobby, big as life, is beaming down at the two of us from a fluffy pink cloud in Paradise. Little wings flutter at his shoulders, and he's wearing only a celestial jockstrap that glistens whiter-than-white. They've restored his health. Not only has he gotten a tan up there, but his muscles are seriously pumped, his hair as brown and glossy as it was in his Florida youth, his eyes as clear and blue as the heavens. He points at us with a wand draped with silvery streamers and tipped with an actual fiery star, and glitter snows all over our sweating bodies and the bed. He approves! He approves! He must have arranged it first thing when he got there. It's six months later in earthly time, but that's as nothing on the Eternal Clock. He smiles and flutters his fingers at us and blows movie-star kisses. We rub at the red lipstick prints on our cheeks with the worn topsheet as he floats off in a shiny bubble like Glinda the Good. Poof! And he's gone—except for a burst bubble, a little asterisk of soap in the air, a whiff of Joy.

The sex, as you might expect after a vision like that—fabuloso. Orgasms for days, both of us literally *howling*. I move in.

Tell us the story of how you got together, our friends beg. It's so romantic. Well, kids, it was like this.

Bobby was positive for such a long time that when he was first tested no one knew what *positive* meant. It sounded so good. He has *antibodies,* I said. I took biology in college. That means he is *fighting it.* They were coming out with these unbelievable statistics from the test, tens of thousands of positives. Some would no doubt develop an immunity. The question was the cofactor: once you were exposed to the virus, what determined whether or not you got the disease?

The race was on to find protection, and maybe it was friendship with me, Amy Hoffman: My friends with whom I ate dinner once a month would never die. Not like that.

Bob got tested because he was participating in a study. He was offering himself up for the good of gay men everywhere, as always.

A man rang his bell once in the middle of the night, a stranger in a city of murders, and Bob opened his door to him, ever generous. He had always dreamed of this, he told him as they embraced. A stranger seeking him out.

Another called him up, interrupting our meal. "Where are you? What are you wearing?" Bob asked. He winked at me and said kindly into the phone, "I'm taking it out for you, man. I'm big and hard."

One sent flowers with a card to our restaurant table, demanding his presence. He left dinner early, ever obedient.

That man gave it to him. And I'll tell, I'll tell his name, because he's dead now, too. That particular, sorry chain of infection is long broken. Ross. Dead and gone. He was Bob's secret affair, terribly exciting, and Ross didn't care about him a bit, not deeply. He had a lover at home, sick, who he would never leave. Bob opened himself to Ross, the orifices Safe and Unsafe. Who knew, then? It was another adventure, another offering.

Finally, and as it turns out, inevitably, Bob was diagnosed.

Full. Blown. AIDS.

Full-blown, like the scarlet amaryllis he forced in January. I hate medical terminology.

At gay pride he was thin, and his hair had gone completely white. He wore a big white hat to protect himself from the sun. He had always done the balloons. Every year he blew up hundreds of balloons. His apartment was filled with them until we marched past his window, which looked right out onto Charles Street, and then he showered us with balloons. He ran up the stairs and danced on the roof. The year of the white hat was the first without balloons. (Since then we never have balloons. We never even march down Charles Street.) He watched quietly from the sidewalk. He waved, but he didn't dance.

Back at home I thought, One day I'll hear that he's dead. I'll turn the page and see his obit. I'll view his quilt. That's why some people cry at the quilt display: They're afraid. They're guilty. They're weeping out of fear that they'll suddenly come upon the patch of an abandoned friend. It will have been stitched by those who did not abandon, who would never abandon.

I ran to the phone and called him up and said I would visit every Wednesday from now on—not that he'd asked for that, but he didn't object. He was a concerned and accommodating guy, the type who picked up stray animals on the street and knew all his neighbors by name.

But before my first Wednesday came around, Bob was in Mass. General, and I visited him there instead of at his apartment. His room was down long corridors, up elevators, on an old drafty floor where everything was green—the walls, the furniture, the nurses' scrubs. The people with AIDS were kept with the elderly, who nodded and drooled in a clump of wheelchairs outside the elevator. The building has since been demolished in a modernization program. It's as though it never existed, nor the things that happened within its green walls.

A nurse directed me to Bob's room, where he was sitting on his bed vomiting a white stream into a basin held by his lover, Steve. Steve sat next to Bob, holding the basin with one hand, stroking Bob's back with the other, his bony back. (I got to know the feeling of his back, which he used to ask me to rub, under my hand, the knobs of his vertebrae, which felt bigger and bigger each week as he lost more weight, the loose blanket of skin thrown over them.) I watched from the doorway, wondering if I should do or say something, until Steve stood up and left to empty the basin. Bob lay down in bed, shivering. This scene between them was private. I should not have stood there.

Ever gracious, though, Bob welcomed me into the room, took my hand in his icy one, and asked me about the weather.

"It's raining out, miserable." I stopped before I said, You're lucky you're not going anywhere. I tried not to be completely stupid. Bob nodded, teeth chattering.

He was so sick. I began to worry about taking care of him by myself. I wrote in my journal, "What if he vomits while I'm with him?"

Would I need to put gloves on to clean him up? What if he choked, too weak to lean over the basin?

Bob's doctor told him the vomiting was caused by MAI, myco-bacterial avium intracellulare, an illness I'd never heard of, because it is an illness of birds. It's bird TB. "I'm Camille," said Bob. "I'm Rima, the bird-girl."

Roberta started visiting Bob daily once he came home from the hospital. She'd go to his apartment after work or early in the morning. She used to shave him, because he found he could no longer stand before the mirror and hold the razor steady. She wasn't afraid of cutting his throat, and she wasn't afraid of his blood. She wasn't even afraid of doing a lousy job. She became his steady hands, his vanity. He'd worn a mustache, but never a beard. I called her and asked, "Shouldn't we take some kind of training to do this? What if he stops breathing?"

"Then there's nothing you can do. Call 911," she said. Now I know —don't ask her a question if you don't want to know the answer, because she'll give it to you. She'll give it to you even if you don't ask. "But don't tell them he has AIDS—they're afraid to come for that."

"What should I tell them?" I couldn't think of even one plausible fib for the dispatcher to explain Bob's collapse.

Later, on Wednesdays, when I would sit in Bob's living room and hear him retching in the bedroom, I would knock and call, "Bob, are you okay? Can I help? Let me in!" and he'd call back, "No! No!" He'd come out of the room after a while, go into the bathroom, then back to bed. I would ask if he wanted another blanket. I'd pile his bed with blankets, but no number of blankets stopped his shivering.

That's AIDS, annihilating even the simplest comforts—a blanket, a cup of tea. I burned Bob with a cup of tea. He took it innocently from my hand and didn't pull away when it was too hot. His re-flexes were fried, even the primal one that jerks the fingers from the fire. Neuropathy. Instead, he stuck to the cup like the peasant who touched the goose that laid the golden eggs and then found himself unable to let go, he stuck to it saying, "Ow, ow, ow," until I realized what was happening and took it from him.

The first Wednesday I visited Bob in his apartment, Roberta was there. I had worried over so many aspects of my visit—calling an ambulance, being a bore or a burden—yet it turned out to be a good day, a charmed day of friendship, the kind of day whose mood I have felt ever since when I walk down Charles Street, especially with Roberta.

She was very sad and angry, because her girlfriend had recently left her after five years. The end had come when they were dressing for work in the morning, each in a hurry and preoccupied with the day to come. Suddenly, an unfamiliar ring of keys had fallen out of the girlfriend's pocket, jangling onto the floor. They lay on the floor between the two lovers—keys to the home of another woman. Not only that, but Roberta's father, who for good reason she detested but who was her father nonetheless, was in the hospital. The three of us talked for a long time in Bob's living room about these problems, Bob sitting in the armchair with a blanket around his shoulders, Roberta on the ottoman at his feet, and me, I don't know where I was. Co-incidentally, my girlfriend had also recently left me after five years, although I didn't say much about this to the two of them, because my true feelings about it were not sadness and anger, but rather shame, for having been in such a bad relationship for so long, and relief.

The three of us went for a walk together—Bob was well enough during those first visits of mine to do that. We ate *gelati* in an Italian cafe, and we browsed through a pile of old photographs in an antique store, hoping to find a picture of someone's dyke aunt posing with her softball team or a nephew in drag. With dusk, it began to snow—soft, puffy flakes. We left with the proprietor, waited as he locked the door, and walked him a half block to his apartment where his boy-friend had dinner waiting.

After Bob died, Roberta and I continued to get together. She was still complaining about her girlfriend, the keyring, and she said, "I can't even make vacation plans. I have no one to go with."

"Come with me," I said. "I don't have a girlfriend, either."

From that point, one thing led to another, to bed and my vision of the Angel Bobby. To true love. The spark is from Bobby. It doesn't fade.

But I don't know about romantic.

I got into an argument with a college buddy of Bob's, this towering butch who he used to visit in Maine sometimes, at the memorial extravaganza, which Roberta organized according to Bob's deathbed instructions — a daffodil given out to every mourner at the church door, recorded whale songs bellowing through the nave, wrenching testimony from those who had fucked him and those who hadn't, the traditional balloon release on the church steps to conclude. Hardly a dry eye in the place. The college buddy got up to the mike and claimed that while Bob was convulsing in the hospital, she was splitting logs with an axe or some such Maine woods chore. Suddenly all the leaves on the tree beside her fell at her feet in a heap. She swears there was no breeze. She believes in this heap of leaves as an actual emanation from Bob's soul as it left the earth. He was fond of nature and trees.

But it was March, wasn't it? Of the proverbial winds? Of the naked gray branches? And the way I heard it, he died in the dead of night.

If it comforts you, okay, I told her, but I only believe in memory. You carry the person within you, and thus he lives, as part of you and yours.

Too bad my memory is full of big holes. Pits, faults, abysses, volcanoes. I knew Bob healthy for ten years, but I only remember him sick. Sometimes I hardly remember him at all.

Maybe I have no feelings. I cried for Bob only once, not at his memorial. I was driving my car when I got a bad headache. Right behind the eyes, a booming pain that spewed up from nowhere. I pulled over and rested my head on the steering wheel. And looking down at my sneakers, I thought, now you know how it feels. If pain and fear started like this — but didn't stop. Bob suffered from terrible headaches. Tears started coming out of my eyes. My pain was nothing like his. Nothing.

Kevin and Me

I was among the guests invited back to Bob and Steve's apartment after Bob's memorial service. Someone had arranged for a dinner to be served. Things got a little out of hand, as they will on these occasions. Every tiny room was jammed with people laughing too hard and trying to manipulate gracefully plates, drinks, napkins, silverware. In the kitchen with my plastic cup of wine I leaned against the refrigerator and watched Tim chatting. Small KS lesions had broken out on his face. He was next. In the bedroom, Richard turned over his plate of lasagna onto Steve's grandmother's wedding-ring quilt and was not forgiven for the mishap. It was past the time to leave.

Then a group of us was sitting in a dark bar, the white napkins under our glasses the only spots of light in the place. "Why aren't our funerals like the ANC's in South Africa?" Kevin asked. He looked around the table at each of us, one by one, but no one answered him. He can get mean when he drinks. "Every AIDS funeral should be a massive protest march." He slapped his hand on the table for emphasis.

Bob died before the real heyday of ACT-UP, before people began chaining themselves to the FDA and blockading the Brooklyn Bridge during rush hour and fantasizing about secret squads of PWA suicide saboteurs — before that guy had his coffin dumped on the White House lawn.

"Protest march against whom?" I said. "To where? It's a virus."

We shouted at each other while everyone else watched, too intent on our fight to be interrupted. I was so angry! It felt great to shout and shout at Kevin and to have him shout back. I wanted to jump up and shake him! He's twice my weight — but I felt like I could wrestle him to the ground! The bouncer had his eye on us. We were about to be tossed out for sure—but suddenly I realized that if I kept it up for another second, I'd start sobbing.

I agreed with him, anyway. I could see his point. This shouldn't be happening. It must be *someone's* fault. It *is* someone's fault. Powerful people up to and including those in the Oval Office must rejoice whenever they hear that our gay brothers suffer and die. That our junky brothers and sisters suffer and die. That our beloved hemophiliacs, babies, Ugandans, Thai prostitutes suffer and die. They must rejoice at it all. They have a serious jones for this news, they slaver for it, they create circumstances in which they cannot but hear it over and over again, it must feel so good to them. They hate us so much.

"I hate gay people," cried Kevin. "Do we ever defend ourselves? Do we avenge our dead?"

We're in mourning.

Don't mourn. Organize!

But who said that? Not someone gay. Not someone from the Age of AIDS.

For a minute, Kevin, can't it be just us? Not hundreds of thousands of AIDS cases worldwide, but just this one person, here in this bed, quietly dying?

Passover

I visit my parents, who are in excellent health—*k'neynehora*—for Passover, and I have a bonding experience with my father over my car, which he has tuned and fixed up, new tires put on, for an exorbitant amount of money that I have been reluctant to spend. The afternoon before the first seder I spend with him driving to the tire dealer. He's pleased I need tires, because tires are something for which he has a connection—we buy them from the son-in-law of his old friend, the late Jerry Bean, who is the father, incidently, of the evil Barbara, a tormentor from my Hebrew school days. Jerry died suddenly of a fast moving cancer, and my father was truly grief-stricken. At the tire shop, he offers Jerry's son-in-law and Barbara the use of our family's cabin in the Berkshires this summer. The son-in-law and my father are both moved by his offer, but can't figure out how to express their emotion in the noisy, gasoline-smelling tire garage, an environment so masculine it's almost *goyische,* which is why my father loves it, he and the son-in-law, two Jewish *shlemiehls,* transacting their business amid the noise and the grease. Puerto Rican teenagers do the heavy work. The son-in-law paces back and forth, then slaps my father twice on the back.

The next day my father insists on taking my car to his mechanic for a check-up, and I end up hanging around the house for the afternoon. My father spends the day calling clients on the phone. He's a salesman, chemicals—flavors and fragrances—these days he's supplying drums of caffeine to soft-drink manufacturers. In between calls, he comes into the living room where I am reading the paper to tell me stories about the people he's talking to and argue with me about the headlines. The Jews, he announces, are evacuating people from

Bosnia, anyone who wants to go, Serb, Muslim, Croatian, the Jews take them all. The Joint Distribution Committee convoys are escaping successfully. It's something we Jews, unfortunately, have learned how to do—whom to pay off, which routes are safe. The UN can't do it.

"Where do you read this stuff?" I ask. "Convoys escaping, the JDC. Why isn't any of this in the *Times?*"

He goes across the street to the gas station to look in on the mechanic. Three times he does that. Finally, the repairs are finished and I leave.

I'm still somewhere in Connecticut dodging trucks and blasting the radio when my father calls my apartment. He tells Roberta to have me call him the instant I walk in the door. He's worried about my safety. The mechanic said the car may need axles sometime.

I dial the phone in the front hall, still wearing my jacket, happy for the chance to please, to obey. I've fallen so far short of his expectations. It must have been over ten years ago, when I was still openly struggling with him and my mother—sending them letters, lending them books, believing I could educate them—that he wrote to me: "I can't accept your lifestyle. I just wasn't brought up that way." And that's been his last word on the subject. Ten years, twelve years, he hasn't budged an inch. (He did not go on, of course, to say anything about *my* upbringing. If pushed, I think he would argue that it was a good upbringing, the best, and that it was only the first of my inborn perversities to reject heterosexuality, thereby rejecting the Jews, rejecting him and my mother. But I haven't rejected them or the Jews. I didn't mean to reject anything.) Our conversation on the phone is exceptionally brief. He answers and says, "You're home? Good." Once he's reassured himself that I'm alive and unharmed—boom— he hangs up.

The previous day, while we waited for the tires, Barbara Bean's husband called her to tell her about my father's offer, then handed my father the phone so he could wish her *gut yontif,* happy Passover. She began to cry.

"She misses her father," my father explained to me when the son-in-law took the phone back.

"I can understand that," I said, looking at him significantly, but he refused to take my meaning.

I meant that I would feel as bereft as Barbara if he died. I wanted him to see that. My love for him.

These days I force myself to imagine the death of my parents, especially when I'm with them, and they're perfectly fine. It's my age, and theirs. The parents of my peers are dying off all around me—not to mention my peers themselves, like Michael, whose father died and left him his VA life insurance, which I inherited when Michael died too, although I never met his father. Earl, his name was. My friends' parents die quickly, they die slowly, they die insane, and with their faculties intact. Like these parents, my parents too will die, and before me no doubt, but they're in such excellent health, despite their age, that the inevitability of it seems more theoretical than real. Even in these times when the deaths of most of the people you see walking around, not to mention that of the entire planet, seem imminent, I can only envision my parents continuing on and on. There's simply no knowing, however many times I try to terrify myself by imagining it, when they'll go or of what causes.

And the question is, would I do it for them? What I did for Michael. I wonder if that was what they were thinking when he was sick. "Don't get too involved," my mother advised me. Was she trying to protect me? Was she thinking, Save it for us.

I'm always wondering what my parents are thinking. I always have a theory, too, and then it was that they were angry at me because they thought I was doing something for him that I might not do for them, my own family. Although actually Mike *was* my family, and I have the paperwork to prove it, the healthcare proxy, the power of attorney, that's what those are about. I did it for him because he was family, and I'd do it for them, too, without question, whatever it takes, moving to New Jersey, cooking, driving the car, changing the bed. My parents are cold to me, and disapproving, but I won't let them get rid of me that easily. I want to ask them, is *this* what's bugging you? Don't give it another thought. We'd laugh with relief. But I can't. They don't like being asked what they're thinking. It's better to try to figure it out.

The risk of giving offense is great, and they show their displeasure—perhaps their pleasure, too—like gods, by not answering, and they can be propitiated only by a reciprocal silence, on that and any other question.

Of course, that might not have been what they were thinking at all. They might not want me there. I do have five other siblings, two of whom live within a half hour's drive and whom my parents have made their executors. What do they know about being executors? I am the eldest and the only one of my parents' six children who has actually *been* an executor, who has purchased a funeral, who has stood in the intensive care unit with the dying—but I've forfeited my precedence. Maybe they think it would make them sicker if I were there with them. Maybe they think it's me with my homosexuality and my sick homosexual friends who is killing them—not with the proverbial heart attack, but rather over the years, by degrees. Maybe they pronounce the word with the accent on the horrifying first syllable, not the second, and they believe I already am. The executor, executing them.

You know, on the holiday we were celebrating, God passed over the first born children of the Jews. Mercifully, He spared them. But the evil children are told: You are as if left behind in Egypt.

The Real Family

So where was his *real* family? My mother would like to know.

Mike's brother, Chuck, mailed him a package during that last week containing a red scarf and a couple of snapshots of his kids. No note. Loie says that when she showed Mike the snapshots and the scarf he moaned, proving that he understood what they were and where they had come from. She propped up the photos on the bed-side table, where he could have seen them if he had been able to look, and hung the scarf over the bed railings next to his pillow. When Roberta visited she examined it with disdain. It wasn't real cashmere, just a polyester blend. Who knows why it was sent — the wife, maybe? "Send him that scarf you got for Christmas, Chuckie. You'll never use it. Boston is cold in the winter." And so it is, my dear, but not in the hospital.

Chuck called me to say he had decided to fly out for the memorial service. He said he wanted to understand his brother's life and why he had become so alienated from the rest of the family. Missed the boat on that one, didn't you, Chuck? What was the big mystery, anyway? Mike's parents stopped writing to him after he came out to them. He was invited to and then disinvited from several family gatherings, in-cluding his mother's funeral, because he refused to promise to lie to the guests. When he was growing up, it was the old story: a bunch of ill-matched people living in too small a space, making each other miserable, beating on the kids. Mike left as soon as he could, and they were secretly just as glad, the big fairy.

On the phone, though, Chuck's voice made your heart stop. He had the sonorous Riegle Voice, the Voice you thought you'd never hear again. Maybe this *wasn't* real, just as you'd always suspected, ever since you read about it in the paper, ever since your first acquaintance died, ever since his diagnosis. Like in one of those pathetic stories my students used to write, it was all but a dream. I had one last night in which Mike appeared at Walta's memorial service, and Freddie too, although Freddie didn't die of AIDS but of esophageal cancer. They were ghosts, but substantial ones, with solid human bodies, and I wanted to avoid Mike the Ghost, but how could I? It was too momentous, his return, and I had to greet him and kiss his rough cheek.

Chuck stood at the back of our small group of mourners, leather-gloved hands clasped behind his back, wearing a camelhair coat and a checked wool cap. My imagination keeps placing around his neck a red scarf. Some, like me, politely spoke to him and tried to make him feel welcome and comforted. We were brought up that way.

The healthy brother, he turns up with his man-of-the-family authority draped about him like a red scarf, and we kowtow to him like deformed trolls living under a bridge to one who walks in the light. The real family doesn't have to do anything, they have merely to exist in their majesty and righteousness, and they are a bulwark to all who gaze upon them.

With AIDS, nine times out of ten it's the fake family who cleans up the shit.

The Angel of Death

Gregory died last Friday in San Francisco. He didn't expect to, even though he was in the hospital with PCP. So many recover from it these days with all the miracle drugs—pentamidine, bactrim. But it had been over a week, and Gregory was not improving. His doctor had a conference with him, told him they wanted to put him on a ventilator to relieve the stress on his lungs, which were almost destroyed because he'd put off treatment for so long. Swiss cheese was what the doctor said. Harry was at Gregory's side, and Gregory turned to him when the doctor left. "Clara," he whispered, using Harry's dear old drag name, "I'm stunned."

When Richard and I talked about it, he said, "I feel like, everybody gets three hospitalizations, and this was only his first, so it's not fair." Gregory thrashed about madly while they intubated him, and for hours afterward, before he lost consciousness, eyes wide open, and died.

He becomes another name on the list of people I've known more or less well who have died of AIDS. I read articles in the newspaper: "Mr. So-and-so has experienced the deaths of 200 of his friends from AIDS." Two-hundred friends, 800 friends, 1,000 friends, a million friends. Reporters cite these statistics with the same pompous credulity and concern for the societal implications—thank you very much—as they did the fabulous numbers of sexual contacts their gay male interviewees used to claim in the late 70s. Meanwhile, in the late night shadows far beyond the media spotlight, Harry says to me on the phone that the memorial service will be a hat party in the Golden Gate Park Rhododendron Glen, which happens to be in glorious bloom this week.

Stupid as the lists might be, I'm not talking anymore to anyone who doesn't have one, who hasn't been ticking off the names of the people they know like they're the *malach hamaves,* the Angel of Death, who flies around with His list. Here's a joke about that from my mother: the 2,000-year-old man, how does he live so long? Garlic. The Angel comes to his door and the man exhales in His face, "WHHHOOO, me?" Of course, for that you need a pair of lungs. *Fuck* everyone who, at the mention of AIDS, wants to tell me all about it because they saw it on TV or sobbed openly at the story of the gallant death of some acquaintance's second cousin. There's a woman who volunteers at the Lunch Place, the soup kitchen where I work, who also works on the Quilt. Her husband, whom she doted on, died suddenly of a heart attack last fall. She's made a life for herself, though, volunteering, writing verse in her spare time. I should admire her. She comes in on Monday mornings and chats to me about AIDS. She went to visit this one in the hospice, to that one's funeral. She goes with the other volunteers, it's like a group outing to the beach.

"It was very sad," she says as we set up folding chairs around the tables. "He was in the hospice for two months. They'll let you stay there for three."

"You can stay as long as you want," I inform her. Wouldn't that be, as Harry says, *the limit*—getting kicked out of the AIDS hospice. I imagine the PWAs in their bathrobes staring blankly at the building, like they sit and stare at the hospice television, only on the street in front of the hospice—actually, there are PWAs living on the street not far from there at all.

She ignores my point, the fact that I, too, know something—know a lot, more than her—about this. "So sad," she insists. "There were a hundred people at his funeral." Like I'd never been to a funeral with a hundred people. Or with ten.

She and I can't comfort each other. She's into her thing, I'm into mine.

Roberta and I went to see a play in New York with her sister and brother-in-law. A man is dying of AIDS. They roll an IV pole and a hospital bed onto the stage. He strips, and his body is emaciated. His legs have that AIDS look—no calf muscles, no buttocks. I wonder, Can they do that with makeup? Has the actor starved himself in a Stanislavskian frenzy? Is he really dying? He stretches his hand around to his behind and pulls it away covered with blood. He screams, and I do too. We see his feverish thoughts. A ghostly Aleph appears behind him and bursts into flame. His ancestors speak. An angel appears above his bed in smoke and thunder. I've sat by the beds of Bob, of Tim, of Mike, of Walta, as they've chattered and writhed, and I've wondered. Flaming angels. I think this is it. Onstage, the PWA's ex-lovers argue about politics in a coffeeshop. Exactly.

Afterward, Roberta's brother-in-law says, "God, was that corny!"

I don't want these people to talk to me anymore. I'm too damn busy. I'm running to the hospital. I'm talking on the phone to California late at night. I'm buying my hat.

Roberta digs up some fifteen-year-old photographs of Gregory posing with others from the old *Gay Community News* staff. He adored being photographed. He placed himself right in the middle of each group. She and I huddle next to each other on the couch, pointing to the men in the pictures: he's dead, he's dead, he's dead.

The Sheltering Tree

It's coming up on a year since Michael died, and Jenifer calls me because she and Loie were talking the other day about organizing a memorial gathering, a *yahrzeit,* a something. They don't want the anniversary to go unmarked.

When I hear her voice on the phone, I don't want to talk to her, but I try to cover it up. She senses my hesitation anyway. As she tells me about their ideas, I act receptive and friendly, until I actually become so, and our conversation grows warmer. I don't have a particular reason for not wanting to talk to her. I like her well enough, but sometimes you pick up the phone, and you wish you hadn't. After Mike died, she and I had dinner together once. Then we called each other every week, then every other, then not at all.

When I hang up I have my assignments: arrange for a place to hold the gathering; contact Fran from the Prison Book Project. But Fran doesn't return my calls.

I always tend toward paranoia.

I suspect that when they were dividing up the names, Loie asked Jenifer to take mine so she wouldn't have to.

I run into Gordon, Rob's lover, twice in one week, first on the street near my office, then on the Orange Line, and I don't think he's overjoyed to see me, although he's one of those gay men with exquisite manners, and we've known each other for years. He hurries off. Rob himself I've never seen, not once. I haven't heard a peep out of him.

We're a group of people who were trapped in a terrible storm. Mike was the big tree that sheltered us. When the rain stopped and the wind died down, we dispersed throughout the woods and fields.

I help with the arrangements, and then at the last minute I call Loie and tell her I'd been planning to come, but I'm just not up to it—although the truth is I'm strong and healthy and generally up to whatever.

The Ceiling

I ran into Carrie outside of Back Bay Station. I'd seen her there twice before, rolling slowly by in her wheelchair, but I'd said nothing.

The first time I didn't realize it was her right away, I guess because I didn't expect a person in a big electric wheelchair that she was operating with her one good hand to be someone I knew—a pure example of prejudice against the disabled. That moment of recognizing but deciding not to go back and acknowledge her stayed with me, and I was troubled by it, but apparently not enough to change my behavior, because I saw her again a few months later, descending from a bus on the wheelchair lift, and even though I'd become conscious in the interval of my bad behavior the first time—and this time I recognized her immediately—I quickly walked past, hoping she hadn't spotted me. I was wearing sunglasses and staring straight ahead, but I thought I felt her glance. I rationalized that I didn't want to get into it with her at the noisy bus stop. I would be saying "What?" "What?" or else trying to fake it through a whole conversation, smiling when she did and nodding my head at intervals. And it had been a long day at work, and I was in a hurry. But not that long, not that much of a hurry—more prejudice.

You know what it is? My family—and I, as trained by them—is guilty of the sin of Sodom and Gomorrah. Which is not, as the *goyim* would have it, faggotry, but its opposite: inhospitality to strangers. We're not helpful, and not only that, we avoid occasions of helpfulness. We don't extend ourselves; we stick with our own. We're punctual folk: no matter what, we keep moving right along to wherever. The other day I was about to go down into the subway, and at the top of the stairs next to me stood a mother with a baby carriage, and I thought, How is she going to get that baby carriage down these stairs? Just then, another woman pushed past me with an angry look and said to her, "Need any help, sweetheart?"

It hadn't occurred to me to offer. I had recognized the problem. I had even felt a flash of annoyance that the transit authority had not installed an elevator at that stop, but once again I'd failed to recognize my role. I've been trying for years to resocialize myself—in fact, the job I was hurrying home from when I saw Carrie was part of that. I was on the staff of a homeless shelter. But obviously I have a long way to go.

The third time I saw Carrie I finally called out. She hadn't seen me, and I had to stand right in front of her chair to get her attention. We ended up talking for a long time, and I easily understood everything she said, noisy buses and all, as though I were wearing the magic hat that enables one to understand the languages of all beings.

People hurried around us to board their buses, and I began to like the image of myself engrossed in conversation with a woman in a wheelchair. I know the most interesting people.

I hate myself. I'm a bitter, hopeless old woman. Hypocritical. Resentful. Selfish.

"I've been thinking about you," said Carrie. "I've been thinking about Michael."

"I've been doing some writing about him," I told her ingenuously, as though I were working on something appropriately tender and nostalgic instead of pissing and moaning and attacking Mike and everything he ever did or said, and all his friends and associates, her included.

"I have too," she said. "There are a lot of things I've had to work through about Mike."

Michael was Carrie's devoted friend for years. We both knew her a little before her stroke—she wrote for *Gay Community News* and volunteered around the office. Whoever heard of a woman in her twenties having a stroke? When she resurfaced two or three years later, from her coma, from the hospital, from the rehab, Michael picked up with her again. He used to visit her every Saturday evening. It was a fine time for him to visit a friend, since his sex life did not revolve around bars or movie dates or a boyfriend who expected the two of them to go out to dinner, but rather could happen anywhere, anytime, but especially on the way home to his beloved Fenway, very late at night.

As Mike got sicker, their Saturday evenings, which by then had been their tradition for years, became sporadic and then stopped altogether. His apartment was three flights up, no elevator, hallways too narrow for maneuvering a chair. He couldn't easily get out, and Carrie couldn't get in. However, a hospital is one place that poses no problems of access, so at the end, when I called her and told her where he was, she came to visit regularly. She thanked me for contacting her and told me she was glad finally to see him.

Then she added that Mike had turned against her during the previous months, that he'd become very angry at her, very nasty. He would call her up and berate her, almost, I imagined, like a breather, some creepy stranger who begins spewing out abuse as soon as you lift the receiver, except, of course, she knew who it was. She didn't go into detail about what he said.

"I had no idea, Carrie," I said. I'd assumed they'd remained friends. I'd imagined long phone calls in which, because of her experience with illness and disability, she had been able to help and support him as no one else ever could.

So I was truly shocked. I got a bad feeling about Michael. I really disliked him. He was always unreasonably critical, but I'd tried to think of this as idealistic, as wanting people to live up to high standards. Until his illness destroyed his privacy, he was a secretive person. Maybe that was what he had been hiding: his meanness.

He was such an asshole.

(Hey! Mike would say, Nothing wrong with assholes!)

I bet it was the old story: He bullied her to prove to himself that someone was weaker than he was. It was a simple matter of brute, physical strength, his against hers. She became nothing more to him than a mechanism of denial. Empathy and good advice were the last things he wanted from her, especially now that they were both, as the mother of a friend of mine once said, *going through the same boat*. He was lost at sea.

Not only did he behave like an asshole to her, his disabled friend, but he had little use for other people with AIDS, either. He'd had one friend with the virus, but they'd had a falling out when Mike brought a trick over to the friend's house for dinner, and the trick stole his watch. It was an old family piece. Mike tried to get the trick to give it back, but of course it was long gone, and the guy denied the theft with the vehemence of a junkie and a born liar. Mike made excuses for him, and that was the end of that friendship. Later, after more than a year of nagging by me and everybody else, Mike joined a PWA support group, but not for long. He said he had virtually nothing in common with the others. A microscopic virus.

"I'm angry at him," I told Carrie. "I didn't realize how angry until I started writing."

But she objected. "No, that's not what I mean," she said. "I know what a jerk you can be when you're in a life-threatening situation. I've been in a life-threatening situation." She drew out the phrase, pronouncing each syllable. "I was a jerk to my girlfriend, even though I wouldn't have survived without her."

"Mike was a very angry person," I insisted. I wasn't as generous as Carrie. I didn't want to forgive him. "Even before he got sick. He was a jerk to a lot of people."

"It's funny," said Carrie. "Other people have said that too. But I never saw it. His humor was wonderful."

His humor! It's not that Mike didn't have a sense of humor. He laughed at the lumbering twists and turns of the powerful, the stupidity of the cat after the mice. But his laughter wasn't easy or happy. It seemed to pain him. He must have been different with Carrie. I wondered what he was like on those Saturday nights, joking and laughing. Not angry. A lighthearted Mike.

Carrie said that during her visits to Mike in the hospital, they made up. "Even in a coma," she explained, "Mike smiled at the names of his friends. He knew it when we came into the room."

And that's where we disagree, and where my anger and bitterness and despair come in. Carrie and several of Mike's other friends think they had some kind of final communication with him as he lay in his hospital bed speechless, occasionally tossing and grimacing. If his eyelids opened you could see that his eyes were rolled back in his head. Even so, if he groaned when they entered, kicked his foot at the mention of a letter received from his brother, moved his head as the loud voice of a doctor came through the curtain from the next bed, they left his room feeling at peace.

"Hang on. Stay with it," Loie would whisper to him, crying and squeezing his hand. She told me, "He knows we're with him. It helps him get through the pain."

Sorry, but I can't believe it. Get through the pain — to where? More pain? Mike wasn't going anyplace. He was just dying, on his deathbed. He had no relationships left, except with pain — he knew no obnoxious doctors, no brothers, no friends. No final reconciliations. No last words. No transcendence. No peace. Just pain and muscle spasms. The worst was when the nurses came in to clean him and change the bed. He screamed and flailed about as they turned him gently onto his side — or, he would have if he'd had the strength. The diarrhea was doing him in. His asshole was an open wound.

"When I was in a coma I went up to the ceiling and watched what was happening down below in my bed," Carrie had said. "I saw the doctors around me, and my girlfriend crying."

"Go to the ceiling," I would whisper in Mike's ear after she had explained that. "You don't have to stay here."

"I've died three times," Carrie told me at the bus station. "It's nothing to me."

She told me she had visited Mike in the hospital on his last day. She'd sat with him and said goodbye, but she left before he died. Sadly, she said she sometimes wonders whether he waited for her to leave him, afraid she would think him weak for succumbing, for failing to find his way back to life as she had done.

But at that point, the virus had sucked up practically every bit of life he'd ever had. Would he still have had guilt feelings, even then? Is *that* what finally remains? I thought one would have moved on to larger issues, but maybe not, maybe that's naive. You are who you are.

Carrie has an authority in explicating Mike's experience that I lack. She's been on the ceiling; I'm stuck down here. It's all I have to go on. She and others have no doubt that their presence at his bedside made a difference to him, a great difference—whereas I sat with him too, every day, but I don't know.

The Teddy Bear

It's the middle of June, six months after Michael's death, and Jacoby invites Roberta and me to dinner. She welcomes us in and immediately begins showing us around the house. We stop in each room while she points out its items of interest. I can tell that Roberta — even though she's perfectly polite and appreciative, nodding and smiling — thinks the place is small, dark, and ugly, and I'm annoyed with her. She's always so sure of her impeccable taste. I'm caught up in Jacoby's enthusiasm, and I think the little rooms are cozy and cute. Jacoby is proud of the home she and her lover have made, and after dinner, to complete the tour, they take us for a stroll around the neighborhood, something we can't do at our beautifully appointed apartment unless we feel like risking mugging or worse. It's an early summer evening, mild enough to be out in shirtsleeves. The weight of the day's heat has lifted and the air is gentle and warm. Jacoby points out the houses where lesbians live.

Back at their house for coffee, she draws my attention to a teddy bear that sits on a window ledge next to the refrigerator. I'm sitting at the table on the other side of the refrigerator, so I can't actually see it. But I pretend I do and don't get up to look.

She says, "This is the teddy bear I gave to Mike. It comforts me every time I see it."

So she's the one who put the teddy bear in Mike's hospital room. I had wondered. To me, he definitely wasn't the teddy bear type: it's a characteristic we shared. Now I find out that to Jacoby, he was. Not only that, but she has no doubt that her presence, even in the surrogate of her bear, eased his pain.

That's what I like and admire about her, and what Mike probably liked and admired too. That confidence.

At the Women's Lunch Place, I had a confrontation with an old woman one Saturday when I was in charge of the kitchen. She came with a carful of clothing to donate just as the volunteers and I were finishing clean-up and getting ready to go home. I went out and told her that I was sorry, but we couldn't accept any clothing donations until the next week, because we'd run out of storage space.

She went nuts. "I'll throw them away, then," she yelled at me. "I'm never giving anything to this place again. I came out of my way to do this. I'm old!" She stamped her foot. "I'm crippled!" She was so angry she was crying.

"Okay," I said. "I'm sorry." I decided I'd better break the rule for her, even though the rest of the staff would be angry at me on Monday when they saw the clothes closet stuffed full of her bags. "I'll find a place for them."

She got in her car and slammed the door and stuck her head out the window. "Forget it!" she screamed. "You try to lead a good life, but it's damned hard!"

After she drove away I laughed at that, but I've been thinking about her. She shouldn't have yelled at me, or maybe I should have yelled at her—but it *is* hard. The homeless women want some cash and a place to live. Mike wanted to feel better. People don't necessarily want the most what you've got to give—lunch, old clothes, a funny little toy.

Or maybe I'm wrong, and they do.

Catherine

I called Richard to wish him happy birthday, and he had a crowd of people at his apartment. He put Catherine on the phone. He loves to pass the phone around. I'd called because usually I celebrate his birthday with him, but this year he didn't come to Boston, instead he had a dinner for himself at home in New York. I thought he'd be pleased that I called. He was, or he said he was, but then he had me mostly on the phone with Catherine, who I've always liked and all, but it's not like she's my best friend, the way Richard is. Or is supposed to be. It's not like it was her birthday. We had a conversation. She told me about her new job, AIDS law. Oh, I thought she was still doing prisoners' rights. She asked about my novel. Nah, it's nowhere. I'm into this stuff about Mike.

I was explaining who Mike was, and she said, "Oh yes, I know who he was. We'd met. I was so sorry when I heard. He was one of the only people who cared about prisoners. Most radicals see them as a little sideshow."

"Prisoners were his life," I agreed.

I was angry all the time, at Mike, at Richard, at myself, at whoever crossed my path, and now at Catherine. She saw Mike as the world saw him. She felt only respect and admiration, while I was immersed in trivialities. I had no idea of his stature or his significance to people. From all over the country, from inside and outside, people wrote to me after his death, mourning, who can take his place? No one. I had filed the letters in my cabinet. Some of them I hadn't even read all the way through.

Six Things I've Inherited

1. A pink flannel nightgown from my mother's mother. It was too big on me, since I was only ten. The sleeves came to my knuckles and the hem dragged on the floor. I wore it to rags. Why I was given such an intimate, homely item at that age I can't imagine, but I loved it. After the funeral, which I wasn't allowed to attend, my aunts said I looked like her. Last summer, for my birthday, my mother gave me my grandmother's wedding ring—when she mentioned that she had it, I asked her for it. She never wore it, but I do, every day. It wasn't a happy marriage. My grandfather was jealous and paranoid and my grandmother a fount of misogynistic Yiddish sayings that my mother occasionally repeats to me, like "every pot has its cover" and "once a woman turns forty you should take her out and shoot her, like a horse." She was sixty when she died from some kind of botched surgery. My mother doesn't explain the specifics.

2. Six hundred dollars from my father's father. He was not a wealthy man, and he stipulated that his legacy was to be divided evenly among me and my five siblings. I dropped out of college and used it to go to Europe with an acquaintance from the Hillel House and a friend of his whom I didn't meet until we were seated on the plane, which gave me the impression that he smelled funny. It was really the recirculated air of the cabin, but we never got along. It was on that trip that I discovered that I hated planes and foreign travel. I had thought of myself as adventurous, but I was terrifically homesick and dismayed by the idea that everyone sitting in the cars in the famous traffic jams of Paris and Rome spoke languages I didn't understand.

3. A Mexican cotton shirt embroidered with a design of marijuana leaves, from Mel Horne. Actually, he gave it to me while he was still

alive and cleaning out his closet, but after he was murdered, stabbed on his way home from a gay bar after closing by a kid who made off with his wallet, it felt like an inheritance. It's not the kind of thing anyone has worn since 1979, but I kept it hanging in the back of my closet for many years. It's now in a box in the basement.

4. The manuscript of Bob Andrews's grandfather's novel, from Bob. Apparently, he had told Steve, his boyfriend, that he wanted me to have it since I was a writer. Steve gift-wrapped various items of Bob's in shiny lavender paper with ribbons and distributed them to Bob's friends after the memorial service. I didn't open mine until many months later, because at the memorial service I really didn't feel like it, and when I did, I discovered that it wasn't the manuscript of Bob's grandfather's novel at all, but galleys of a notorious gay male S/M novel, *Mr. Benson,* with Bob's comments penciled in the margins. How Bob came to have those galleys and why he wrote comments on them no one will ever know. As it happens, I actually met the author of *Mr. Benson* at a party — he's died since then — and I told him of Bob's possession, and consequently of mine, of the galleys of his masterpiece, but although he was flattered to hear about Bob's admiration for his work, he could not recall ever meeting him or giving him anything. I didn't read the book — I often find pornography embarrassing — but Roberta did with great enjoyment. Eventually I told Steve that he had given me the wrong manuscript, and he wrapped up my correct inheritance, which once again I didn't read and Roberta did. Or rather, attempted to. Grandfather wasn't much of a stylist, and Bob did not chose well in designating me guardian of the Andrews family's literary heritage. I threw it out the last time I moved.

5. A dark red, handwoven chenille scarf, also from Bob. I wear it as I type, along with my grandmother's gold ring. Steve got into giving away Bob's things, every time you saw him he had a package for you, and one day I met him and Roberta — this was before she and I got together, when she was just a person I knew — in a restaurant, and he gave me the scarf. He had accompanied Roberta on a shopping trip for furniture. She had bought a couch. As we seated ourselves, she asked, "How do you deal with your grief if you don't go shopping?"

I didn't know what to say, because I was in graduate school and couldn't afford much. I thought that probably — certainly — I wasn't dealing with my grief.

Although gifts and inheritances are so often disappointments, the scarf is something I would have chosen for myself. It's soft, pretty, and wraps around me warmly with the original owner's presence. I like to think I remember Bob wearing it with his black leather jacket — now Roberta's, her inheritance — but the truth is that I don't know for sure that I ever saw it on him.

6. Mr. Earl Riegle's veteran's life insurance settlement, plus miscellaneous cash, from Mike Riegle. Isn't it strange how, as one's gay family supersedes one's birth family, the gay family, that is, me, becomes the keeper of the birth family's legacy. I'm thinking of Bob's grandfather's novel and Mike's father's (pathetic) life insurance, and how I, a middle-class, second-generation, Jewish lesbian from New Jersey inherited from two redneck old men whom I never met, and who would have been outraged to know their male progeny had made me their heir. (To whom will I leave my grandmother's ring? Certainly it could go to one of my nieces, but perhaps it would be more in keeping with the pattern for the adorable Lily Wen Rui and Mei Lin Dan to fight over it, the Chinese adopted daughters of Berit and Betsy — full name Cornelia Elizabeth, the third or maybe fourth since the ancestral Cornelia — my old friend and one-time lover.)

Mike left everything he owned to me and made me his executrix, but his written will didn't tell the true story of how he wanted his assets, such as they were, distributed. This he told me privately, and I wrote it down and dated it when I got home. After he died, and I'd paid the cremation costs out of his savings, I sent checks for the amount he had left, half each to the Prison Book Project and to *FagRag*, as per his instructions. I only learned about the life insurance after that, when his brother turned up at the memorial service. He told me there would be something, not much, about $1,500, coming to Mike, or rather, his estate, and indeed he sent me some forms to fill out a few months later, which I did, eventually receiving and again distributing the check. *FagRag* hasn't put out an issue in at least five years, even with Mike's money, and Prison Book waited so long to deposit their legacy that when they did, it bounced, and when I wrote them a new check they once again didn't deposit it, and I had to go in person to Stephanie's apartment on South Huntington Avenue and practically beg her to do it, and the whole incident royally screwed up my account so that in the end I think it cost me.

Two Dreams

1. Mike is alive, although sick. Roberta and I are sharing a house with him and a group of radical fairy gay men. He is good in this dream, gentle and reasonable, and later, telling Roberta the dream, I say, "I don't deserve to be visited by a good incarnation of Mike, after what I've written."

The house is under siege. A man speeds by in a pickup truck and begins firing bullets at the house. He is a big man with a rosy complexion and a mustache, wearing a white cowboy hat. A macho guy. (I didn't describe this man to Roberta. There's always a piece you leave out when you tell a dream.) Luckily, the bullets don't hit anyone. They hit the floor, digging a deep groove into it. The man laughs and drives away.

We decide to go to the police. Everyone in the house piles into cars. I think Mike will naturally oppose this idea of the police, but he agrees with everyone else that our situation is dangerous, and we have to try everything. He and I jump into the same car, along with Roberta, who is clearheaded and practical and makes me feel safer, like there is a way out.

When we get back, the man with the white cowboy hat is there, with accomplices. This time, they drop bombs on the house, but these also luckily don't hurt anyone. They are more like a warning. When we pick them up from the ground, they are peas. (Similarly, I had picked up the bullet that had been fired at us to examine it, and it was a bullet-shaped piece of wood.) But then the men come with a bulldozer. We are in the house terrified that they will collapse it around us. But the bulldozer isn't powerful enough for that; it splinters some wood at a corner of the house, but mostly it tears up the ground and trees outside.

The dream is getting more and more frightening, and I want to wake myself up from it and hold onto Roberta, but I can't. Then the alarm rings, and I jump up to get ready for work.

I usually believe that only the dreamer herself can interpret her dream, but Roberta must explain to me that this dream is about AIDS in our lives. We are with gay men. They are sick, and no one will help us. We are terrified. Our community, our "house," is in danger, besieged, although for now it is strong enough to stand. But who knows what they'll come back with after the gun, the bomber, and the bulldozer?

2. One night, as I undress for bed, the snapshot of Mike that I've propped up on the bookcase catches my eye. He is posed so naturally and his expression is so much what his was that it's hard to believe the picture is not of a person who resides in this world, moving around and expressing himself in his characteristic manner.

He visits me later in my dream, wearing the same shorts and tee shirt he's wearing in the picture.

"Touch me," he says, sitting down next to me, knowing I think he is a ghost.

I reach out to his thigh, and his thigh is real—I feel the hair, the flesh and the bone—and my hand does not pass through it as through a mist. He is not dead. He has proven it to me.

Walta's Birthday

I come home from Bronski's house with gifts: a home-baked pear torte missing one slice, a book I've been wanting to read, and a form letter he's written that I can copy and send to ten of my friends urging them to vote for rent control. It's Walta's birthday, the first since he died, in honor of which Bronski had promised to change the message on the answering machine and get his hair cut, but when I arrive he hasn't done either of these things.

He says maybe Monday.

Personally, I don't mind the answering machine, but it drives some people nuts: Walta's voice is still on the tape, with one of his beloved divas shrieking in the background. There was a night, near the end, when I was visiting, and Bronski decided to bring Walta into the kitchen. To lift him, Bronski would sit him up in bed, feet on the floor, and stand in front of him. He would bend at the knees and place Walta's hands on his shoulders. Then he would say, "Okay, here we go," and rise, lifting Walta upright. Arranging Walta so he stood between the two of us, one arm around Bronski's shoulders and the other around mine, we kind of dragged him over the threshold of his bedroom into the kitchen. The three of us sat together at the table, Bronski and I yammering away, Walta slumping farther and farther over in his chair. He'd said nothing since I'd arrived, just glanced up at me from the bed when I came in, with that terrified gaze he'd taken on, his eyes cavernous and dark. At the table he looked horribly uncomfortable, and I felt it was wrong for Bronski and I to go on talking around him—a parody of the evenings the three of us had spent together at this table, yelling for hours about books and music and politics, Bronski and Walta running around the apartment and pulling books down from the shelves to reinforce their points. A record was playing, something gorgeous and sad. "What is this?" I asked. "It's beautiful."

"I'm not sure," said Bronski. "I just threw it on the turntable."

Suddenly Walta looked up. "Leontyne Price," he mumbled. " 'Marietta's Lied' from *Die tote Stadt*." And he began to hum along — a quavering, almost inaudible vibration.

This is what is left. Always something.

Bronski caught my eye. "My boyfriend," he said. "He can barely walk or talk, but he could be a contestant on Opera Quiz."

Bronski admits it's been three years since his last haircut — he and Walta used to go together — and his hair is down to the middle of his back. He pretends it's a secret vow, a gift to the gods, who in all that time haven't shown much appreciation. Roberta thinks Bronski's ponytail looks ridiculous, and she is not alone in this opinion — she's also anti-answering-machine — but I'm in favor of it, it's so seventies, just like Bronski himself, when he and Walta met. 1974. New York City. The Club Baths.

He and I go out to the back porch, although it's October and chilly. The sun is out, and after some time it warms us. Walta used to sit on the back porch in all weathers, smoking. Two years or so before this, it was August, Roberta and I had been visiting him. He was sitting on the porch wearing a beautiful blue-and-white striped cotton robe, which he suddenly stripped off, exposing himself. "Is this okay? Is this okay?" he kept asking, and we said of course, the sun was hot, we knew him well. He was so demented.

Later, the doctors discovered, totally by accident, that his confusion was being caused by a build-up of fluid in his brain. They had hospitalized him for a spinal tap in another attempt to diagnose his problem, and when he woke up, completely lucid, he said to Bronski, "I feel like Chinese food, how about you?" Surprised that they'd developed a successful treatment, the doctors continued to drain the fluid periodically, and Walta improved for a time — he began writing poems again, listening to opera and Nina Simone, reading, keeping a journal. (Many months later, after he had stopped reading and writing for good, I sat in the wooden chair next to Walta's bed reading a manuscript of his poems that Bronski had compiled. Walta had written the poems, but he could no longer read them. "These are your poems," I explained. "You are my favorite poet." He looked at me, terrified.)

Before the memorial service Bronski gave me Walta's journal and asked me to pick out some passages to read. I was honored by the request and then surprised to find that the journal was almost entirely about smoking and how ashamed Walta felt of it. He wrote that he had no self-control. In the old days he used to smoke a special brand of cigarettes called Fatimas—they're discontinued now, and even then he could only buy them in a special shop in Harvard Square—just one or two in the evening. He kept them in a silver case that he would bring out after dinner, and he lit them with wooden matches from a tiny cardboard box laminated with a picture of a white swan.

On the porch Walta chain-smoked Camel straights. During his good times, you'd find him out there reading or writing or entertaining other visitors. Later, he'd be hunched way over in his chair and smoking, although he'd usually look up and say hi when you sat down.

I sit in Walta's chair and Bronski sits in the other one, but he immediately says, "Why don't you sit over here, the sun is stronger," and we switch.

Bronski remarks that last night David came to dinner. David's birthday is exactly the same as Walta's. They were even born in the same year. The birthday is not exactly the same, Bronski says. Walta was several hours older.

The porch is full of plants that are flourishing beautifully despite the chill and the fact that plants were something Walta did, while Bronski affected not to have the interest or skill. But they've been watered, pruned, repotted, fed by someone. I'm eating a slice of freshly baked pear torte—Bronski's always done the cooking—and drinking tea. Bronski asked, "Do you want lemon?" and I said "No, just sugar," and before pouring the tea he took the sugar shaker and held it upside down over my cup letting sugar stream into it unmeasured, exactly the way the homeless women used to do it when I worked at the shelter. "Stop! That's too much!" I said, and he spooned some out. The tea is delicious. I can never get it to taste like this at home.

Bronski tells me his news: he's angry at Chris. He claims to have yelled at Chris on the phone, although I find that hard to believe, since I've never known Bronski to confront anyone openly, no matter what awful things he's been saying behind the person's back. It's unfortunately true that Bronski's sentences often begin, "So-and-so is my best friend, *but.*" Chris was supposed to go out with Bronski this evening, the evening of Walta's birthday, but another friend offered Chris a theater ticket, and he left Bronski a message on the answering machine, not even bothering to reach him in person, saying he had decided to do that instead, even though Bronski was getting them tickets to the same show—it gets a little confusing. Bronski says, "Chris is my best friend, *but*" and lists many character defects: he's emotionally immature, unreliable, withdrawn. "Chris spends as much time as he can by himself. But I'm not like that. I loved living with Walta and having our friends around."

I don't know what to say.

Bronski's words become tangled like smoke among the plant leaves. He's no longer living the life he loves, although he used to. He's so lonely. There's no cure.

Mike Eating

Mike's friends gather for a yearly memorial to him, the second, a potluck dinner. Most of those attending worked with Mike on the Prison Book Project, and they invited everyone to spend the afternoon with them beforehand, fulfilling prisoners' requests for reading material, as Mike would have done.

I helped organize the potluck, but I didn't want to go. I allowed myself to think I wouldn't, even as I was throwing together a casserole, putting on coat, boots, scarf, hat, mittens. Michael died in January, and this year on the anniversary there are two feet of snow outside. My body aches from shoveling. Some of the guests can't make it because they have the flu. At least there are no remembrance rituals involved in this event. We just eat and talk.

It's actually kind of nice. I'm liking everyone there and feeling sorry I didn't make myself help with the mailing in the afternoon, when Fran announces that Prison Book is eight months behind, and they've decided to stop sending out science fiction and the like and to concentrate instead on essentials like dictionaries, legal information, and *The Autobiography of Malcolm X*. Mike would have been pleased. He was annoyed by requests for novels, didn't consider them serious. Fran urges us to donate our old copies of the autobiography, and any other books of interest we might own, since we are of an age to have read them years ago and to be unlikely to open them again. We can always get them from the library or even repurchase them if we must.

I happen to own not only *The Autobiography of Malcolm X*, but a collection of his speeches and a biography. And it's true that I first read the autobiography decades ago, but I reread it not long ago at all. I started the biography too, but it was very badly written. I had found it on a remainder table. I've never yet opened the speeches —

but I might. I'm proud of my little Malcolm reference library. I don't want to give it away. I like owning books, rereading them, looking things up when I forget them. Even if I don't read them, I like knowing they're there. Fran pushes. "Your old books would be really appreciated by guys in the joint." Of course she's right. I volunteer to call publishers and try to get books for free.

Carrie is passing around photos of a prisoner Mike used to correspond with, whom she corresponds with also. "Where did you get these?" someone asks, and she explains that the prisoner isn't allowed to keep more than a certain number, so that when he gets a new photo, he has to give an old one away, and he's been sending them to her. "That's not such a bad rule," Terry says, just as I'm thinking about how egregious and mean-spirited it is. "I mean, to live by. Getting rid of old possessions before accumulating any new ones. Of course, in prison it's different."

It's all very Mike, who famously despised possessions. And yet he accumulated them compulsively, hated to throw away a thing. He hung them on his walls, crammed them into his closets, piled them on the floor. He had a drawerful of old pill bottles, another of shrunken tee shirts. Things like that. Candle stubs. A chair with a broken rocker. Sticks, shells, and leaves he'd collected outside. Letters, books, inspirational quotations, and pictures of cute boys cut out from magazines. And all over everything, notes to himself on yellow Post-its. "Wear underwear," said one that he'd stuck to his alarm clock where he'd see it in the morning. He'd been having trouble controlling his bowels, and briefs provided a little extra protection in case of an accident. Before AIDS, he'd preferred to go without. They seemed unnecessary. A rebel right down to his skin. He explained this to me—"You know I hate wearing underpants"—when he drew my attention to the note. He was in the hospital, and he'd asked me to go over to his apartment to pick up some things for him. He thought I'd find it funny, but I didn't. I found it infuriating and pathetic. Because of his stupid habits but also because of the way his illness inhibited them.

Terry ought to know perfectly well what Mike was like, since he helped clean out the apartment after Mike died, which transmutated his things instantly into meaningless junk that needed to be put in black plastic bags and hauled down to the Dumpster. I don't know what Terry's place is like, but Mike's was no monk's cell. Except for his kitchen, which was spare, uninhabited. After Fran's announcement we go back to eating and talking—two things Mike did, in company, steadily and persistently, until he'd gobbled vast quantities, or held forth for a good hour at a time. Yet he thought of himself as abstemious and silent.

He had the mental attitude of a bulimic, if not the behavior, despising food, yet craving it, needing it of course, yet despising his body's pleasure.

"The food here is great," says Carrie. "Mike would have loved this."

"Except nobody brought dessert," someone points out.

"That's true. Mike loved dessert," Carrie says. "He used to eat a pint of Ben and Jerry's when he came to my house. Once he ate a whole box of cookies I'd been saving." She laughs, enjoying this reminiscence of Mike's foibles. The others laugh with her, but her story leaves me fuming.

None of them seem troubled by the hypocrisy of Mike's relationship to food, how he would have shoveled down Carrie's ice cream and cookies, not allowing himself to taste them. He didn't believe food was worth paying for. He stole it, and he periodically got caught. He hung around hoping you'd invite him for dinner. For himself, he felt he had better things to do with his money. He was a moocher.

"But he would never have bought those things for himself," I say to Carrie, wanting to make her see.

But this makes her laugh even more, and the others, too. "Oh, I know," she says. "That Michael!"

And there I sit, raging over something that everyone else remembers with affection. They did know what he was like. And yet, they didn't mind it at all. They loved it.

Why are my feelings about him so much less straightforward than everyone else's? For me he was so difficult, for them so easy. I probably knew him for the longest time, although not by much. He'd apparently told me bits of personal information that he kept from others. When Carrie suggests that next time we gather on his birthday instead of on the anniversary of his death, I'm the only one who knows when his birthday was. In the old days at *Gay Community News,* Richard, Michael, and Jil all had May birthdays, one each successive week, and Mike's was last. He wouldn't celebrate with cakes or parties; he would spend the day alone reading *King Lear.* I know that, too. In the hospital he asked for Shakespeare, but the collection Rob brought was too heavy for him to hold. He needed one play at a time, in small paperbacks—but then, he could no longer focus on reading. I wonder if we should read from Shakespeare at Mike's birthday gatherings. Not likely. It's too much a luxury of Western civilization. When I wrote his obituary, friends of his called to talk to me: this one hadn't known about his degrees, that one his languages, the other his piano playing. But I knew it all.

Mike and I had started out by working together every day, in that intense little place, amidst deadlines, political disputes, love affairs, threats from the outside world. On the night after the office burned down, we did our shift together, watching in the alley in case the arsonist came back. I was friends with him, one way or another, for thirteen and a half years, from the night we met—when he came to volunteer for layout, and the two of us were sent out together to buy the beer because neither of us had any other useful skills—until the night he died. That first night, I walked with him through Beacon Hill. He was wearing his Greek fisherman's cap, his expatriate years in Italy just recently over. He was newly out in the United States.

He kept his friends apart from one another, preferring to enjoy each relationship separately, and there were always people popping up whom I'd never heard of before, but whom he considered tremendously special. It never occurred to me until just now, this minute as I write, that maybe I was one of those special people too, that he looked forward to seeing me, too, and deliberately chose me to confide in.

He loved me. The idea is new and strange. Did I love him? Yes. No question. (Although through everything, over all these years, I've rarely put it to myself like that.) From the very beginning I saw him, Michael, in all his Michaelness, and I never lost sight of that no matter what, and I think that is love. So, maybe he was glad when I turned up and said I was there to take care of him. At the time, I didn't think he took my offer seriously. But he must have been relieved. He knew I was the type to come through. As angry as I got at him, as frustrated and upset, it didn't occur to me to stop, and he knew it wouldn't, and gave me his love and trust. He never said that—love—and I didn't much either, for a lot of reasons. But there it is.

Mike's Dick

At a dinner party, for reasons known only to my hostess, I'm presented to this guy named Larry as one of the *Gay Community News* staffers from the old days—like I haven't done anything since then—and as I'm shaking his hand, he says, "Oh yeah? *Gay Community News?* I used to trick with the tall guy. Up in the bathroom there." It's not the first time I've been introduced to Larry, our paths have crossed before, but apparently women don't register too clearly on his screen. He's that kind of gay man. To be fair, he was high the other times I met him, and this evening he's on the wagon.

"That's Mike! He used to trick with Mike!" several of the guests say excitedly.

"Mike," says Larry. "He had a bent dick. I still remember that, it was quite unique. It went at like a 45 degree angle."

"Well, that's something I never knew," I say, ever polite. Although I'd seen Mike exposed. In his last days, cleaning him off when he shat himself.

"You wouldn't," says Larry. "Not unless you saw him with a woody."

Everyone in the room is looking at me significantly. "Hey, Aim, this is great! This has to go in the book!" I've become known as a Mike specialist, a Mike collector. As I write, I create him, and he's mine, all mine, all his deeds and effects. I think of his body. I flash on it decomposing horribly in its coffin, the busy dick, however it was made, bent or straight, long gone. He was forty-eight. It's been two and a half years. Then I remember of course I had Mike cremated. I and his friends scattered his ashes in the Fenway Victory Gardens, his favorite tricking place, and there is no coffin, no body in the ground, and I'm so relieved.

That night I dream. I was in the old *GCN* office, the one that burned down, that Larry remembered. Mike was there too, and a couple of other people, although their identities were kind of fluid. They were more recent staffers. They didn't know Mike or me very well, and they went about their business without paying us much attention. Mike was sick. We were in the old office, but we were also in a hospital, and I wanted to take him to this special room they had where he could lie down and nap. But as in so many of my dreams we became lost, and a place that had seemed simple to get to became mired in complication. I dragged Mike up staircases and along corridors, as he became more and more ill and pale and exhausted. Then a nurse, or someone, said we couldn't go to that room anyway, because it had become contaminated. There was a disease in it, and it was cordoned off and quarantined.

Maybe after that we were in the office again, and Mike lay down on the green couch. But also our fruitless and exhausting wandering continued on and on — until the dream fades away. I fall into a deeper sleep or more likely wake up in a sweat. Even in dreams I make the wrong decisions and exacerbate the worst situations.

No rest for the weary. That was Mike's motto. Chuckling, he repeated it often. Sometimes he said, "No rest for the wicked," instead. He is ashes, but his body persists in memory: weary, wicked, wandering. Bent and delicious. I don't give him any peace, dragging him around like this.

Conclusion

Kaddish

Everywhere I go lately I hear the kaddish. It's all over the news, the latest thing. They had a rabbi chanting it in a movie I saw, and also in a play on Broadway, a garbled version, but I knew what it was. I used to be a good Jewish girl, a scholar. Even now the Hebrew words cry out to me with beautiful meanings. Holy. Merciful. Peaceful. Many times blessed. Amen, amen, amen. The Jews believe in life, life goes on, my mother explained to me when I was ten, and her mother died, and as testimony to this faith, she has since refused to acknowledge the going on of anything but. Life. Since then, I have never seen her cry. The kaddish is a prayer of reconciliation, she said. Of acceptance. I accept the universe! proclaimed the transcendentalist Margaret Fuller — whom the City of Boston has memorialized with the elementary school across the street from my apartment, children laugh and cheer in the playground as I write — and Carlyle quipped famously, She'd better. The bitch. But I won't. I won't. Accept this suffering, this order that encompasses it, this karma, this harmony of the spheres. You won't catch me saying a kaddish over anyone's remains. It's not for me to join in praise of the Named One, Who in His Wisdom named for us AIDS.

Amy Hoffman is a writer living in Boston.

Urvashi Vaid is the author of *Virtual Equality: The Mainstreaming of Gay and Lesbian Liberation.* She lives in New York City.

Library of Congress Cataloging-in-Publication Data
Hoffman, Amy.
Hospital time / by Amy Hoffman; foreword by Urvashi Vaid.
    p.   cm.
ISBN 0-8223-1927-6 (cloth : alk. paper). —
ISBN 0-8223-1920-9 (pbk. : alk. paper)
1. Riegle, Mike — Health.   2. AIDS (Disease) — Patients — Biography.
3. AIDS (Disease) — Patients — Hospital care.   4. Caregivers.   I. Title.
RC607.A26R5364   1997
362.1′969792′0092 — dc20   96-35144
[B]